How to Die Young at Ninety

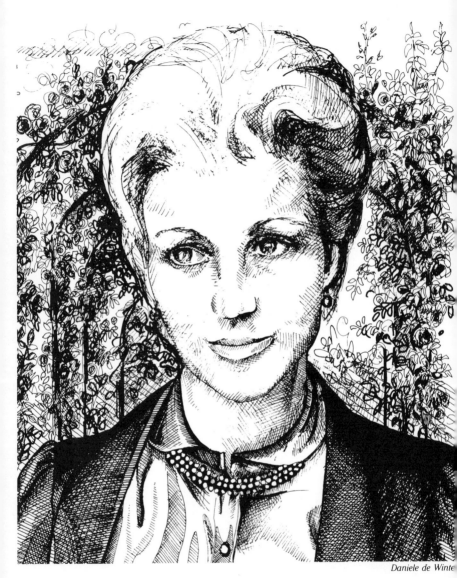

Daniele de Winte

The art of living consists of staying young in mind and body
when no longer so in years.

Dr Jan de Winter

HOW TO DIE YOUNG AT NINETY

A Blueprint for High Quality Living

Printed in Great Britain
by
Manton (Westminster) Ltd
Foredown Drive Portslade
Brighton
and bound by
The Newdigate Press Ltd
Dorking Surrey

First Edition 1982

Published by
The Dr Jan de Winter
Cancer Prevention Foundation
6 New Road, Brighton, BN1 1UF

ISBN 0 9507511 1 1

The Author gratefully acknowledges
the help of
Carol Fisher for the illustrations
Daniele de Winter for the design
and artwork for the book jacket and
for the illustrations
Vida Herbison and Jenni Balow for
kind permission to publish the excerpts
Carol Robinson for the typescript
Gerald Burkeman for editorial work and layout

To the memory of

MICHI

About The Author

Vida Herbison writes:

"He's a charming man" said a friend when she knew that I was going to see Dr. Jan de Winter at his home in an ancient downland village. "Although he never says anything about it", she continued, "I know what he thinks and I have to admit he's right, but it always makes me feel guilty".

My friend is a heavy smoker and Dr. de Winter, for more than 30 years in Sussex, has not only worked to cure cancer but is a prime mover in this and other countries in endeavouring to educate the layman in its prevention.

As he spoke I realized that he was one of those rare people who seek not only to help by precept but also by his own example. The result is obvious. He looks bronzed, fit and far younger than his 67 years. He originally came to England from his native Austria for six months in April 1939 to perfect his English but the war intervened and he volunteered for the RAF.

In 1950 he took up his post as Senior Consultant in charge of cancer treatment at the Royal Sussex County Hospital, Brighton. Dr de Winter's international reputation grew and over the years he contributed to three major text books on the subject of cancer as well as numerous other scientific publications.

During his work in Sussex he has cared for more than 20,000 terminal cancer cases. In 1967, after years of campaigning and thanks to the generosity of one of Brighton's most respected families who donated their mother's old home, Copper Cliff, and with the aid and encouragement of the late Lord Cohen, and Lady Cohen, he was able to found a long-term nursing home for cancer sufferers. Here the 22 patients each have their own room and every comfort. Dr de Winter remains the Honorary Physician in charge.

Dr de Winter also visits most schools and colleges in Sussex where he gives talks to Sixth Formers in an endeavour to get them to understand the function of their bodies, how they could be harmed by misuse, and how, by sensible living, they can avoid cancer in later life. He advocates personal hygiene, the right diet and exercise. His ideas, he says, are not always popular because when one is young one likes to experience everything in life. Disease and death (especially from self-inflicted causes) can seem so very remote.

Dr Jan de Winter is by no means a puritanical health fanatic but he advises everything in moderation because the human body is an exquisite masterpiece and should not be abused, as most of us in the modern world tend to abuse it. His book "How to Avoid Cancer" sets forth clearly and optimistically just that. It is wittily illustrated and the jacket cover, designed by his daughter Daniele when she was only eighteen, shows remarkable originality, imagination and sophistication. The book may be obtained on application from the Dr Jan de Winter Cancer Prevention Foundation, Freepost, Brighton BN1 1ZZ. price £5.

In September 1982 Dr. de Winter will open a High Street Clinic for Cancer Prevention Advice, (the first of its kind in the UK) next to the Theatre Royal in Brighton, where anyone on an impulse may walk in and ask advice.

After meeting Dr. de Winter, I must admit that even I try to live sensibly. Just as my friend said, he does tend to make you feel guilty and in my case it's because I know he's so right.

CONTENTS

Author's Foreword

The main aim of this book is to highlight the vital link between nutrition and correct weight in the avoidance of premature ageing and degenerative diseases.

In the affluent West for instance, one person in three eats too much and too richly; as a result one person in four is seriously overweight and periodically attempts to redress the situation by intermittently submitting to one or the other of the 600 listed slimming regimes, only to regain the lost weight on resuming the old eating habits.

Apart from looking less attractive and being at serious risk from degenerative illnesses, an obese person has the added disadvantage of ageing more rapidly. The reason for this is simple: a person is as old as his or her arteries. Since the condition of one's arteries hinges on the degree of self-imposed moderation and restraint, clean arteries, like a clean driving licence, are achievable only by constant vigilance and in the absence of habitual indiscretions.

For instance, of the twelve different categories of environmental factors, dietary factors are estimated to contribute up to 37%, smoking 30%, sexual behaviour 7% and alcohol 3% to overall cancer mortality. Thus three out of four cancer deaths are known to be due to self-indulgence and are therefore avoidable by a change in personal habits.

Many illnesses are thus brought on by the wrong sort of food and drink that we consume compounded by such bad living habits as lack of exercise, stress and smoking. This causes the arteries to become clogged-up, the blood-stream to become sluggish and the tissues to become oxygen-depleted.

By contrast, free-flowing blood in clean, elastic arteries is the best insurance against illness and premature ageing, with diet as first line of defence and exercise as a second line.

However the novel art of living that this represents will be unacceptable to most adults who have grown up with the mistaken belief that, for instance, only animal proteins have any "goodness" in them, that potatoes and bread are more fattening than meat and fats or that cold food is less nutritious than hot food. In other words, before they will be prepared to accept fruit, vegetables and cereals as their staple diet, in preference to meat, fats and confectionery, a fundamental change in traditional and inherited eating habits will have to take place.

This change will have to go hand in hand with a much wider range and much greater availability of quickly prepared, high-fibre, low-fat and low-sugar-content foods, which will be sold in new take-away salad bars, which would compete for customers with "fish and chips" shops. Similarly, "fresh fruit-holding slot machines" would provide an alternative to the currently so very popular processed and prepacked convenience foods, which abound in (empty) calories, that is they are almost devoid of nutritional value.

The case for anticipatory care is nowhere better proved than in the prevention of such degenerative diseases as cancer, heart disease, high blood pressure, strokes, diabetes and obesity. To wait for these diseases to develop is bad medicine. The "rule of halves" indicates that for every patient identified to have the disease there is another in the community about to develop it. Therefore, the earlier the underlying dietary and other contributory causes are detected and corrected the greater the chance of avoiding the disease altogether and with it premature ageing, thereby also, very importantly, preserving individual freedom and independence, the two precious personal prerogatives which are so essential for, and conducive to, meaningful enjoyment of life.

West Dean, 1982   Jan de Winter

THE ICEBERG OF ILLNESS

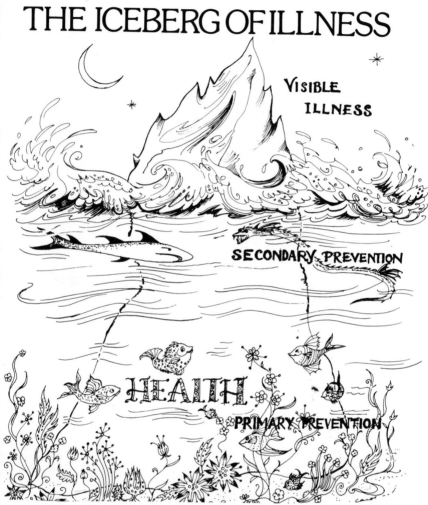

The three complementary medical systems in use against the three-tier *Iceberg of Illness* are: 1. Orthodox conventional treatment for established, (visible) illness. 2. Secondary prevention, that is prompt detection and cure of early disease, and 3. Primary prevention, that is, maintenance of health through avoidance of known predisposing factors.

Introduction

Unless the doctors of today become
the dieticians of tomorrow,
the dieticians of today will become
the doctors of tomorrow..
Alexis Carrel

Many of today's disabling illnesses could be avoided if only we could learn to temper our habitual weaknesses with discretion and restraint. Yet even this simple precept, because it tries to achieve better health at the expense of self-indulgence, is too vexatious to be generally acceptable in our hedonistic consumer society.

This book, therefore, is addressed particularly to the health-conscious few who are prepared, perhaps even eager, to learn in good time how to avoid illness and enjoy a high quality of life well beyond the eighties, something for which our body tissues are admirably equipped because they can keep living almost indefinitely. When tissues degenerate they do not degenerate because we grow old — we grow old because we make them degenerate by the way we live. Body-tissue-breakdown, like the breakdown of a high quality car, is mostly due to bad driving and poor maintenance.

15

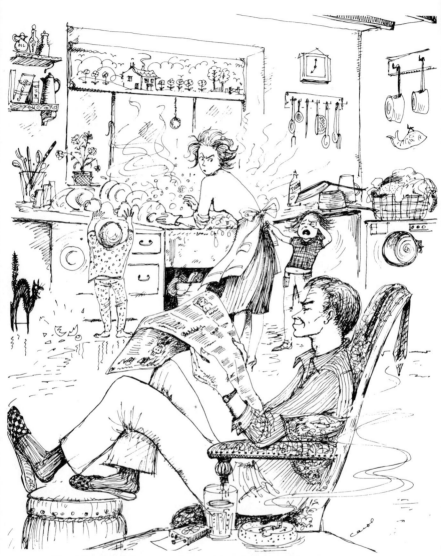

Good health, like a good marriage, is extremely vulnerable and therefore in need of constant care; if disaster is to be averted, thoughtless practices must be eliminated.

This remarkable capability for high quality survival depends on the condition of our arteries; we are as old as our arteries and their condition depends entirely upon temperate living. Clean arteries without fat-deposits, like a clean driving licence without endorsements, are achievable only by constant vigilance and in the absence of habitual indiscretions.

In this respect, as in others, good health is uniquely akin to a good marriage: both are delicate, both are vulnerable. To thrive they need endless care and loving attention. Nothing is more likely in the long run to erode good health, or a good marriage, than repeated thoughtless practices. So if disaster is to be averted, these must be identified and eliminated quickly.

Some Chapters end with a list of questions specially formulated to reveal to the reader whether his or her particular mode of life includes potentially dangerous personal habits likely to contribute towards contracting one or more of these degenerative diseases.

Though formidable in number, these are largely self-inflicted and therefore avoidable. They include heart disease, hardening of the arteries, high blood pressure, strokes, liver cirrhosis, obesity, gallstones, diabetes, breast cancer, bowel cancer, cancer of the cervix, chronic bronchitis, emphysema and lung

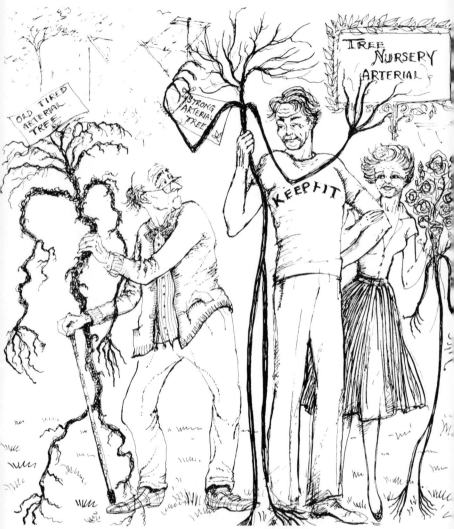

A person is as old as his or her arteries. When, as a result of sloth and gluttony, arteries get clogged-up and the bloodstream becomes sluggish and oxygen-depleted, tissues are starved of oxygen and laden with waste products, which hastens degeneration and ageing.

cancer, but it should again be stressed that these illnesses are largely avoidable.

Although heart disease claims most lives, it is common to find symptoms of other degenerative diseases simultaneously with it. The main cause of these illnesses is a sluggish, fat-clogged, oxygen-depleted bloodstream which is a result of the sort of food and drink we consume, combined with other bad living habits such as lack of exercise, stress and smoking. Conversely free-flowing blood, in clean and flexible blood vessels, is the best insurance against these degenerative diseases with diet as a first line of defence and exercise as a second.

Main Causes of Death

Cancer
1/4

Heart
Disease
1/3

Strokes
1/6

Daniele de Winter

Other Causes

75% of all deaths are brought on by the wrong sort of food and drink we consume, coupled with such bad living habits as lack of exercise, stress and smoking.

Diet

All these illnesses, though common in Western countries, are rarely found in the less sophisticated parts of the world. Yet even in Western countries most of these degenerative diseases have become widespread only during the last sixty or so years. It follows that the main causes must lie in some aspects of our modern way of life and it can be shown that most of them are related either directly or indirectly to what we eat.

There are two main reasons for eating; of these the first is concerned with the provision of nutrients, for tissue growth and repair, for muscular activity and for chemical reactions in the body.

The second reason, rarely conducive to good health, but for many a more pleasurable one is that we eat for *fun*. Since we eat food, not nutrients, we need to know which of the three main types of food i.e. proteins, fats and carbohydrates are most required for good health.

Proteins

These are to be found mainly in meat, fish, dairy products and cereals. In fact, proteins are the only

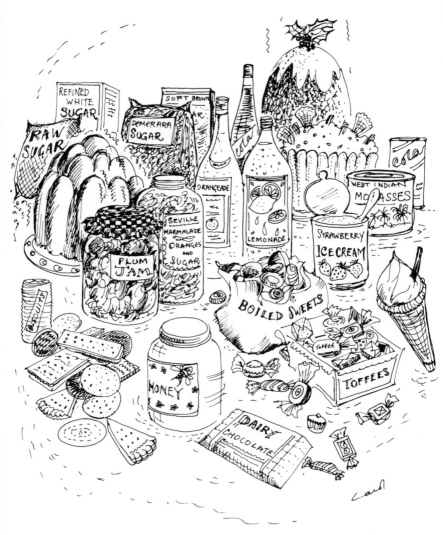

Sugar is totally without nutritional value in whatever form it is taken, whether as white sugar, brown sugar, raw sugar, Demerara sugar, molasses, syrup, honey, jam, marmalade, orangeade, lemonade, biscuits, chocolate, sweets or ice-cream.

really essential nutrients because they are needed for tissue growth and repair and since the body is unable to synthesize them, about 10% of our food intake should be in the form of proteins.

Fats

The most commonly eaten fats are butter, margarine, cooking fats, salad oils, mayonnaise and dairy cream. *All* fats are not only unnecessary but can actually be harmful, particularly when eaten to excess.

Carbohydrates

These are comprised of

1. **Sugars**, which are simple carbohydrates

2. **Starchy foods**, which are more complex. Starchy carbohydrates such as wholemeal bread or potatoes provide some of the important dietary fibre required for the proper functioning of the intestines and are thus essential for good health, but *sugar* is totally without nutritional value *in whatever form it is taken* — white sugar, brown sugar, raw sugar, Demerera sugar, molasses, syrup, honey, jam, marmalade, orangeade, lemonade, Cola, cakes, puddings, biscuits, chocolate, sweets or ice-cream — what we are actually eating is *sugar,* chemically pure but full of fattening calories.

VITAMINS

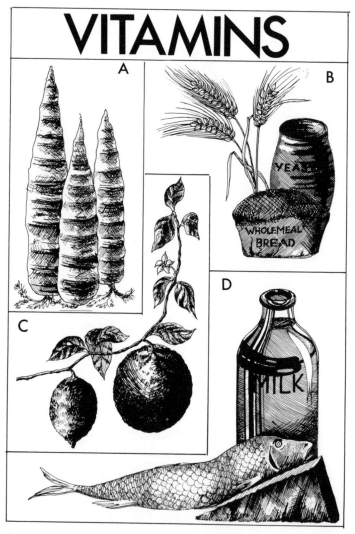

One carrot contains a 3 days supply of Vitamin A. Vitamin B is found in cereals, yeast and pulses (beans and peas). Half an orange contains a 1 day supply of Vitamin C. Milk and cheeses are rich in Vitamin D, as are fat fishes.

This refined sugar, it must be stressed, is completely unnecessary for good health because the little the body needs is amply supplied in a simpler and healthier form in fruit and milk.

Vitamins and Minerals

No-one eating a mixed diet of proteins, starchy carbohydrates, vegetables and fruit should need any vitamin or mineral supplements in tablet form.

In any case one carrot contains a three day's supply of Vitamin A which is also plentiful in yellow fruit and green vegetables. Well-fed people have about a two years' supply of Vitamin A in their livers.

The Vitamin B complex, consisting of half a dozen different vitamins, is found in cereals, yeast and in pulses (peas, beans, lentils).

Half an orange contains one day's supply of Vitamin C which is also found in fresh fruit and vegetables.

Milk and cheeses are rich in Vitamin D, as are cod-liver and herrings.

All of the most important minerals are plentiful in a mixed diet and so there is never any likelihood of a shortage. They include: calcium (found in milk and cheeses), phosphorus (contained in poultry and sausages), magnesium (present in bran and nuts), iron

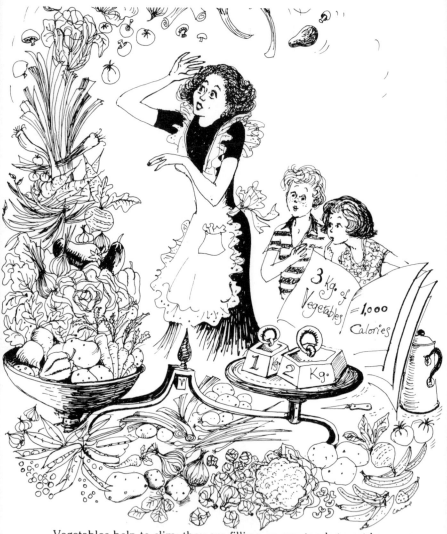

Vegetables help to slim: they are filling, so one tends to eat less;
being rich in dietary fibre, they help to combat constipation.
Being low in calorie content, they can be eaten freely.
Nutritionally all they contain is Vitamin C.

(contained in curry powder, red meat, liver and baked beans) and zinc (present in meat, offal and shellfish).

Fruits and Vegetables

Apart from containing Vitamin C, fruit and most vegetables have no other appreciable nutritional value, but being rich in dietary fibre, they are filling and so tend to reduce appetite and the risk of obesity.

Even more important, they are bulky, and by promoting active bowel peristalsis, help to reduce constipation.

Rice

Rice (preferably brown rice) should be cooked in a pressure cooker in as little water as possible in order not to leach out the Vitamin B. The water should not be discarded but used for cooking.

Potatoes

Potatoes, a starchy food with 2% protein and 80% water, contain Vitamins B and C. It should be noted that the Vitamin C is destroyed when:

  a. potatoes are cooked in a copper vessel

  b. they are kept hot for a long period

  c. they are re-heated

  d. the water in which they are to be cooked has not been boiled first to remove the oxygen

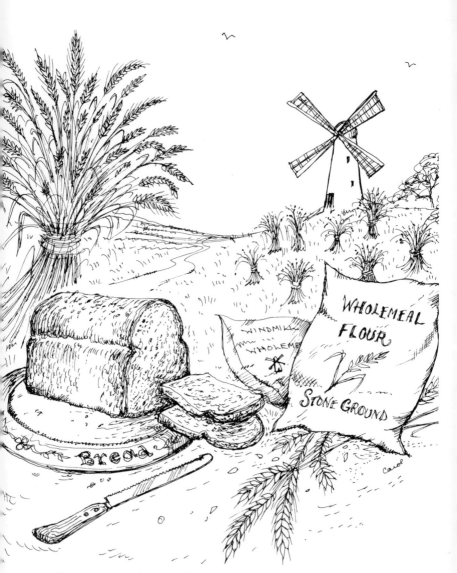

Only bread made of wholemeal flour contains 100% wheat grain as well as fibre-rich bran; because it also contains 10% protein, it is nutritionally an ideal food.

e. they are cooked in too little water, which encourages the presence of oxygen

f. they are cooked with baking soda

It should be emphasized that potatoes are not fattening provided that they are boiled, or baked and eaten in their jackets without butter, oil or margarine.

Bread

A standard 500g loaf contains 250g of starch, 50g of protein and 10g of fat; the rest is water. It is often called a starchy food, which of course it is, but it also provides an adequate amount of protein — in fact from the point of view of *protein* we could live on bread alone. Bread made of wholemeal flour contains 100% wheat grain of which 8.5% is fibre, whereas bread made of white flour has lost 30% during milling and thus has only 70% of the wheat grain and no fibre-rich bran at all. Yet white bread continues to capture 90% of the market sales and wholemeal bread only 1%! Brown bread with 0.6% of fibre is second in popularity, capturing 9% of the market.

Excess fat and sugar consumption

Much of the serious ill-health prevalent in our over-fed third of the world is self-inflicted, since it is caused by excessive consumption of fat and sugar.

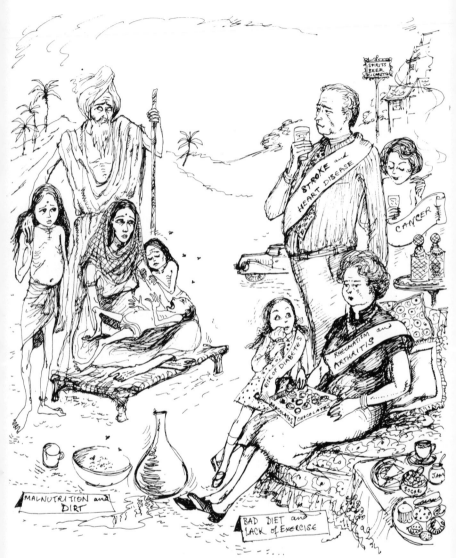

Deficiency diseases of the poor and ignorant in the starving East are matched by degenerative diseases of the affluent and the ignorant in the overfed West.

It is surely extraordinary that Third World Communities, so far not affected by the degenerative illnesses of the sophisticated West, should strive so desperately for the greater affluence which will bring in its wake the same toll of Western ill health! What a sad reflection on the lamentable state of public enlightenment in the West that in the last quarter of the twentieth century, the *deficiency* diseases of the *poor* and ignorant in the East are matched by the *degenerative* diseases of the *affluent* and ignorant in the West.

The enormous increase in the 20th century of degenerative diseases in the sophisticated communities is unquestionably due to Western eating habits. Not only do we eat double the calories needed but compared with the under-privileged nations we consume 7 times as much fat, 6 times as much sugar and about 10 times as much cholesterol, whilst we eat very little in the way of starchy or fibre-rich foods. During both World War I and World War II degenerative diseases in food-rationed countries decreased, as they also did in prisoner-of-war camps and concentration camps. These beneficial dietary effects, which were most pronounced in meat and dairy-producing countries (where land-use was changed to grain production) can be attributed to the complete absence of fat in the meagre war-rations.

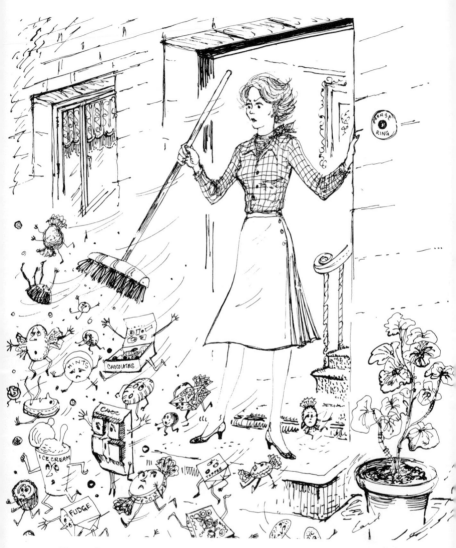

Never have sweets in the house. Sugar and fats are needed as a source of energy solely for heavy physical activities. Even for superbly fit people there is no dietetic "carte blanche" which would allow them to eat excess fats and sugar with impunity.

Fats and sugars are needed solely as a source of energy for heavy physical work and for athletic pursuits. In the absence of such physical activities regular excessive intake of fat and/or sugar will inevitably lead to fat storage and weight gain. This is why 40% of the Western population are over-weight and 30% try, unsuccessfully, to slim at least once a year and in the process they spend annually £40 million in the UK and £350 million in the USA on slimming cures.

Even for superbly fit people there is no dietetic "carte blanche" which would allow them to eat and drink with impunity because they soon lose the low blood viscosity and high blood-flow velocity character-istic of athletes, which affords such remarkable protection against degenerative diseases.

Few people realize that 10% of most sweetened soft drink is composed of sugar; that alcohol drinks are fattening; in fact that 20% of the calories eaten in a day come from sugar and almost 40% from fat.

Roughage

Neither sugar nor fat contains any dietary fibre whatever. In other words they have none of the high-residue roughage contained in wholemeal bread, bran, breakfast cereals, pulses, fruit and vegetables. This means that at least 60% of the food-energy eaten

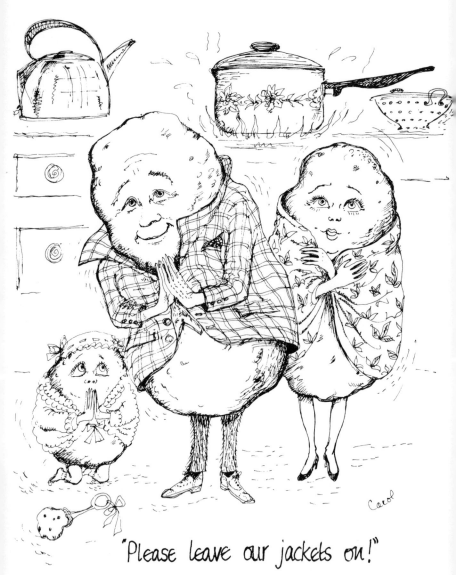

"Please leave our jackets on!"

Fibre-rich starchy potatoes baked in and eaten with their jackets are not fattening, provided they are consumed without butter or margarine.

34

every day is totally devoid of roughage even though dietary fibre is the *only* component of food with a low calorie content and therefore not fattening.

Obese people, as well as looking less attractive, have a higher risk of developing degenerative illnesses like diabetes or heart disease, so there is every good reason to strive to stay slim. This can best be achieved with the help of fibre-rich food because a substantial part of it remains unavailable for digestion and so decreases (by 2%) the amount of food-energy that is actually absorbed. The indigestible portion is expedited as unabsorbable roughage straight through the bowel. As a result of its heavy bulk it easily provides the 200g of roughage necessary to trigger off the emptying reflex in the rectum, and because of its soft consistency it is much more rapidly excreted, thereby combating constipation and with it, a host of other illnesses. Additionally, its bulky volume increases and prolongs the "full-up" feeling and reduces the desire for food. For instance high-residue, fibre-rich wholemeal bread is much more filling than soft, fibre-depleted white bread, white cake or white biscuits. This is also the reason why fibre-rich, starchy potatoes (either boiled or baked in their jackets) contrary to general opinion, are *not* fattening, provided they are eaten without butter or margarine, and not cooked in oil.

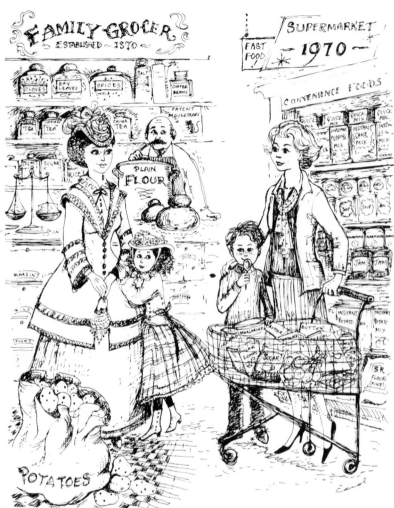

In 1870 80% of our food-energy came from wholemeal bread and potatoes and 20% from sugar and fats. One hundred years later 60% or more of our food-energy comes from eating fats and sugar and less than 40% from cereals and potatoes. It is this dietary reversal which is responsible for the alarming increase in degenerative diseases in the latter half of this century.

Most people have been brought up from infancy almost exclusively on low-fibre, high energy foods containing much fat and sugar which lead to many degenerative diseases. Fortunately today there is widespread awareness that a high-fibre diet is both healthy and slimming.

Despite this, when it comes to changing lifelong eating habits, few can bring themselves to forego the old accustomed over-indulgence in the wrong kind of food and drink.

So it must be emphasized again: bran, unrefined cereals, wholemeal bread, whole wheat flour, unpolished rice, vegetables, fruit, fish, poultry, skimmed milk and low fat cheeses should be eaten regularly because they do not clog up the arteries. What should be *severely restricted* or *avoided altogether* is butter, cream, fatty meats, fried food, unskimmed milk, high fat cheeses, mayonnaise, ice cream, sugar, confectionery, cake and alcohol. All these foods have a high fat and/or sugar content. This increases blood viscosity and slows down blood velocity and so pre-disposes to tissue breakdown, premature ageing and a poor quality of life.

Because of the health-promoting effect of food rich in dietary fibre it is particularly regrettable that the daily wholemeal bread and potato consumption has

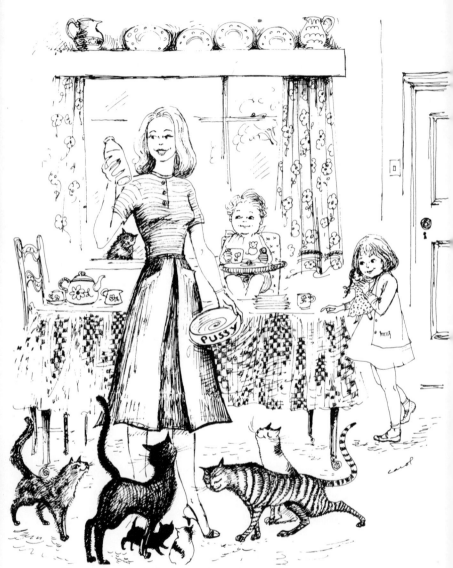

Since cream is fattening and can be harmful, the top of the milk should always be given to the cat.

been severely reduced. In 1870 it averaged 400g of wholemeal bread and 300g of potatoes (providing a daily total of 40g of fibre, 8g in the form of crude fibre). By 1970 it had dropped to only 200g of *white* bread and 200g of potatoes (yielding a total of 10g of fibre, no more than 2g in the form of crude fibre). This is exactly one quarter of the dietary roughage eaten one hundred years ago.

The ill-effects of such fibre-depleted diet are compounded by the concurrent reversal of the relative proportions of fats, sugar and starches that are eaten today. Whereas in 1870 only 20% of our food-energy came from sugar and fats (the remaining 80% being provided by cereals and potatoes) now 60% or more of our food-energy comes from eating fats and sugar and less than 40% from cereals and potatoes. The increasing incidence in the 20th century of diet-related degenerative diseases in the overfed third of the world is a direct consequence of such uninformed and undiscriminating food selection.

This adverse trend is readily reversible by a simple change in dietary habits exemplified for instance by a switch from whole milk to skimmed milk (or always giving the top of the milk to the cat!) or, by habitually having fruit or low-fat yoghurt for a dessert instead of pudding, cake or fruit-pie.

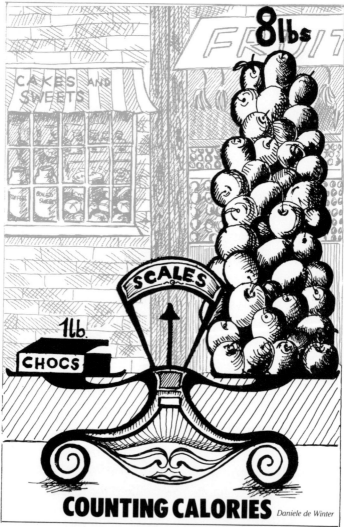

COUNTING CALORIES *Daniele de Winter*

Chocolates contain by weight eight times the calories of raw apples which means that the caloric content of a one pound box (½kg) of chocolates is equivalent to that of eight pounds (4kg) of raw apples.

Calories Consumed

In practice the only effective method of controlling one's weight is by counting calories. Calories are measuring units which indicate the amount of energy contained in an item of food. A few practical examples might aid better understanding: we consume 100 calories by eating either 1 slice of bread and butter, or a ¼lb of spaghetti, or a ¼lb of haddock; 1 whole water melon, or 1 banana; 2 cauliflowers, 2 cucumbers, 8 lettuces or 10 tomatoes. Similarly we absorb 100 calories when we drink a half-pint of beer, a glass of wine, a small sherry or a single whisky. In addition alcohol may stimulate appetite. Sweets contain by weight, six times the calories of boiled potatoes and eight times the calories of raw apples, yet they are completely devoid of nutritional value.

The calorie content of food can be readily calculated: Each gram of fat yields 9 calories, each gram of alcohol 7 calories, each gram of protein and each gram of sugar 4 calories respectively. From this it is very obvious that fat has the highest calorie content per volume and that eating butter and margarine, or constantly frying foods in cooking fats or oil will immeasurably increase calorie absorption; a percentage of these surplus calories not needed to fuel the body with energy is then stored as body fat and this is what makes people overweight.

41

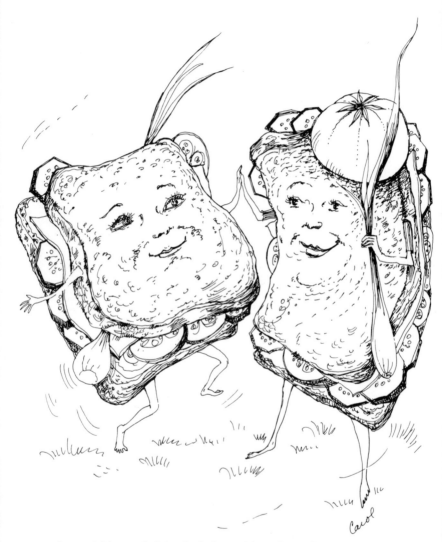

A vegetable sandwich of wholemeal bread supplies not only far fewer calories than a cake or other confectionery but by virtue of its bulk it will promote intestinal peristalsis and combat constipation — something a piece of cake can never do.

Constipation

Because of its vital importance to health, it is worth repeating that eating vegetables, fruit and high-fibre foods, will not only supply far fewer calories but by virtue of their bulk will tend to prolong the "full-up" feeling thus reducing appetite and promoting intestinal peristalsis. This is very important because constipation is still one of the commonest disabilities in the affluent West and aperients remain in such great demand that each year £4 million are spent on laxatives in Great Britain and £35 million in the USA.

Calories Expended

Calories are used, not only to calculate energy *absorbed*; they also serve as units to measure energy *expended*. The simple effort of merely staying alive requires a non-stop energy supply for all the biological processes taking place in the body.

For instance, in any one day, calories are required for over 100,000 heartbeats and for more than 60,000 breaths.

Calories are expended to keep the brain functioning and to maintain the continuous snake-like peristaltic movement of the bowel. They are needed to keep up the body temperature and used on the exchange of fluids as they pass in and out of the body cells. Even in bed, calories are consumed at the rate of one per

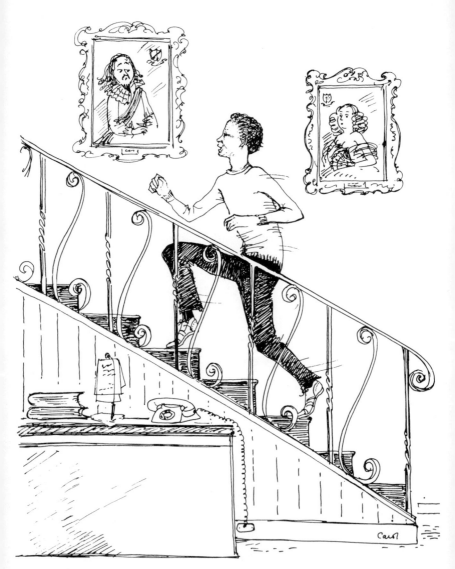

Whatever your age do not use a lift. Always run upstairs, preferably two steps at a time, thereby expending 20 calories a minute.

minute: nearly 500 are used up in a night of 8 hours sleep.

Muscular activity however, requires by far the most calories. We use 2 calories per minute when sitting and writing; 3 when driving a car; 5 when walking quickly or polishing a floor; 7 playing tennis, 10 digging or shovelling, 11 cycling fast, 14 swimming vigorously and 20 a minute when running upstairs.

The average daily calorie requirement for an active adult male is thought to be in the region of 3,000. The greatest consumption, as would be expected, is during the 8-hour working day, when half of the total is used. The 8-hour leisure period needs another 1,000 calories and finally, about 500 are used up during the night. It is interesting to note that for an active adult female, the figures are lower. She requires only 2,300 calories and consumes 1,000 at work, 900 at leisure and 400 at night.

Weight Gain

It is not unusual for some women to gain about 20kg (44lb) in the 20 years between the age of 35, when the average weight is 60kg (132lbs), and 55 when it is 80kg (176lbs). How imperceptibly this increase comes about will be more readily understood when it is realised that *one* extra slice of bread and

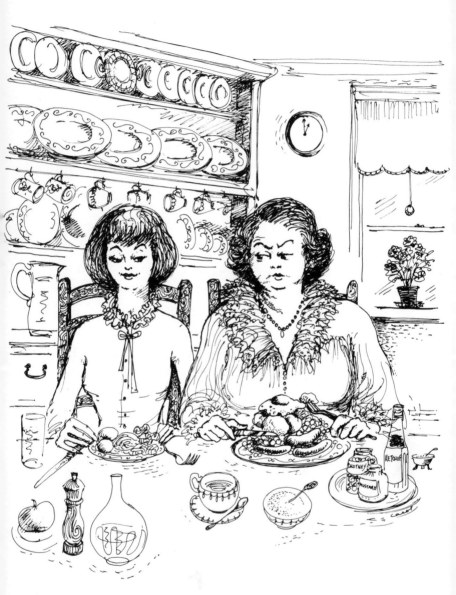

When one uses a small plate one tends to eat less.

butter a day can contribute an extra 100 calories a day. This represents an extra weight gain of 3 grammes a day and repeated daily this will work out at more than 20 grammes a week or 1kg (2lbs) a year. All this from only one extra slice of bread and butter a day!

If one continues to eat the same amount of food year after year one will gradually gain weight as one grows older because with age the body requires less energy to satisfy its metabolic needs. Additionally, physical activity usually decreases after young adulthood and if the food intake remains constant, the resultant weight gain will also be constant. Because of the serious risk of obesity to health, life insurance companies charge over-weight people much higher premiums; from their actuarial records it appears that the life expectancy of a person who, at the age of 45 is 12kg (26lbs) over-weight, is reduced by 25% and that he or she is likely to die at the age of 60 instead of 80.

It should be emphasized that it is infinitely simpler to maintain weight than to try to lose it once gained. As an example: to lose 1kg a week, the total daily food energy intake must be reduced by at least 1,000 calories and this requires tremendous motivation and a will-power of iron. To be more specific, to lose 1g of fat the food intake must be reduced by 7 calories;

47

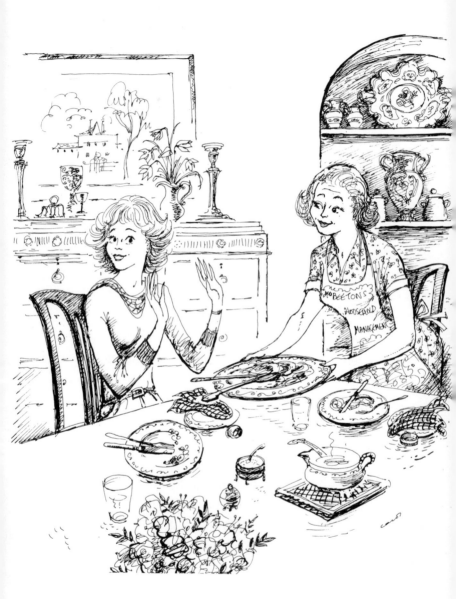

It is a sound rule never to accept a second helping.

therefore, if the desired weekly weight loss is to be 1kg (and it is unwise, and invariably unsuccessful in the long run, to attempt a more rapid loss of weight) the usual food intake must be cut by 1,000 calories a day. Such drastic reduction in energy consumed results in a daily loss of 150g. If maintained every day this will result in a loss of 1kg in a full week.

So to lose weight it is important to count the calories in *every* item of food. A tablespoon of mayonnaise, for instance, has more than twice the calories of a tablespoon of pure sugar and a tablespoon of ketchup has about the same number of calories as a teaspoon of sugar.

Questions on Diet
(Any answer in the affirmative is favourable)

Do you eat fruit regularly

Do you have lashings of vegetables

Do you take unprocessed bran every day

Do you buy only wholemeal bread

Do you prefer poultry to red meat

Do you eat much fish

Do you cut off all visible fat

Do you prefer your meat boiled (steamed)

Do you avoid fried or roast food

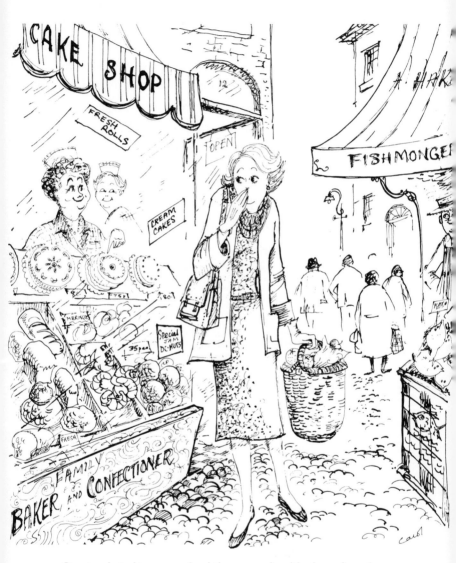

One tends to buy more food than one should when shopping on an empty stomach. Therefore always shop after, not before a meal.

Questions on Diet — contd.

(Any answer in the affirmative is unfavourable)

Do you take your tea or coffee strong

Do you take butter

Do you take cream

Do you drink whole milk

Do you eat more than 4 visible eggs a week

Do you take sugar

Do you eat chocolates

Do you eat rich creamy desserts

Do you have more than one main two-course meal a day

Are you constipated

Are your stools small and hard

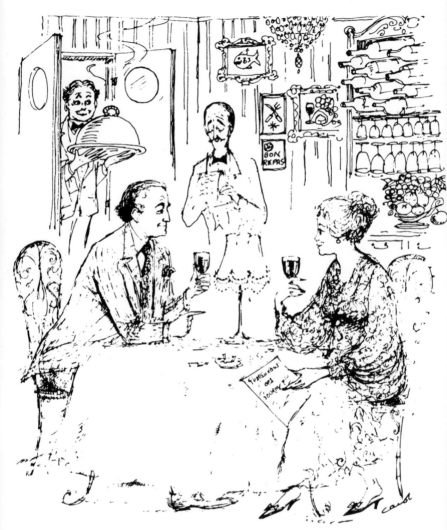

An aperitif, three glasses of wine with a meal and a small liqueur or brandy afterwards total 650 calories which is equivalent to having eaten a second meal. To expend this extra food energy in physical activity would require a brisk two hours' walk or 60 minutes of strenuous cycling or a 40 minutes' fast swim.

Alcohol

Excessive alcohol consumption is known to contribute to liver cirrhosis and cancer as well as to premature loss of sex-drive and brain atrophy. It is frequently forgotten that alcohol is a high-energy food which passes straight through the blood into the fat stores. There are over 70 calories in a half-pint of beer or a small glass of sherry, 90 calories in a glass of wine and 130 calories in a single whisky.

It is not unusual for the average person when invited out, or sometimes even when dining at home, to have 2 single or one double whisky before a meal, 3 glasses of wine during a meal and a small brandy after a meal. This relatively moderate amount of alcohol adds a total of 650 calories to the food consumed, which is equivalent to having eaten a second meal.

This additional energy, if it had to be used up, would necessitate 2 hours brisk walking or 1 hour of fast cycling or 45 minutes of energetic swimming, for without this physical exertion these 650 calories would inevitably be converted into a weight gain.

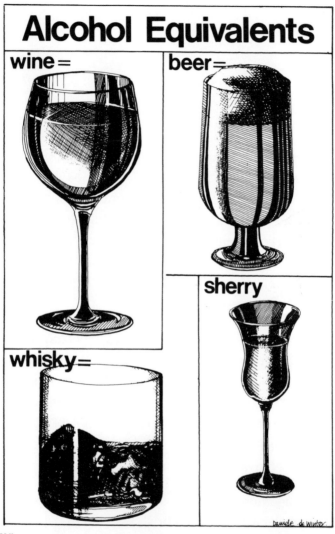

What matters as regards alcoholic drinks is not the type of drink but its alcohol content. Half a pint of beer is equivalent in alcoholic content to one small sherry, or one glass of wine, or a single whisky or gin.

There are five important guidelines which should govern the amount of alcohol that can be safely consumed:

1. The type of drink is irrelevant.
2. What matters is the alcohol content of the drink.
3. Half a pint of beer is equivalent in alcoholic content to one glass of sherry or wine, or to one small whisky or gin.
4. Three pints of beer (or its equivalent, that is six glasses of wine or sherry, or six small whiskies or gins) if drunk at once is too much because it not only raises the alcoholic content of the blood above the legally permissible level for driving but also because if taken regularly it will eventually lead to alcoholic dependence.
5. Four pints of beer (or its equivalent in alcoholic content, that is eight glasses of wine or sherry, or eight small whiskies or gins) when taken regularly inevitably damage one's health and must eventually lead to addiction, that is chronic alcoholism; an "occasional binge" does little harm.

Immoderate consumption of alcohol is particularly damaging if it is associated with cigarette smoking. The two seem to interact, i.e. each potentiates the effect of the other and can often cause cancers of the mouth, pharynx, larynx and oesophagus. These diseases are found more frequently in men employed

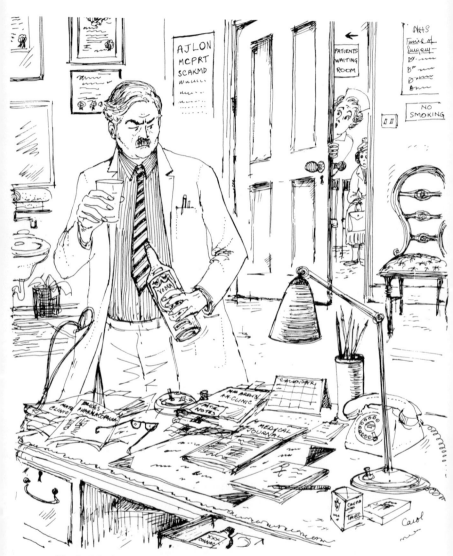

Alcohol induced illnesses, particularly liver degeneration leading to fatal liver cirrhosis, affect all social classes including the medical profession.

in alcohol-associated trades such as the French vineyards, the cider-based liqueurs industry in Brittany and Normandy, in publicans and in employees of spirits and brewery enterprises.

Alcohol-induced illnesses, particularly fatty degeneration of the liver leading to fatal liver cirrhosis, affect all social classes including the executive ranks of business and the professions, especially the medical profession.

Questions on Alcohol:
(Any answer in the affirmative is unfavourable)

Have you drunk alcohol for 10 years or more

Do you feel a regular need for alcohol

Do you drink spirits

Do you take wine regularly

Do you need alcohol to raise your spirits

Has your appetite decreased

Do you feel nauseated at times

Do you sometimes actually vomit

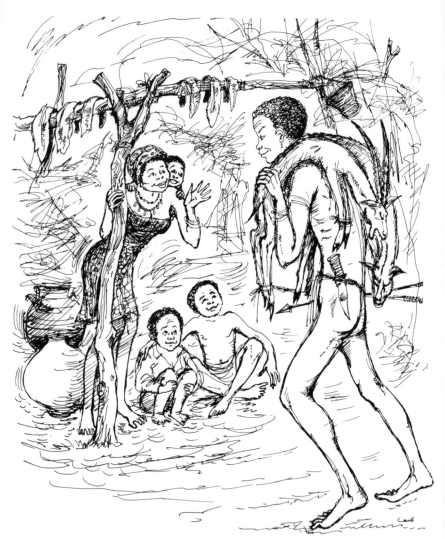

The Kung Bushmen of Botswana who are still separated from civilization, are slim because they hunt for their food, they have no tooth decay or diabetes because there is no sugar and they have no heart disease because their diet is fat-free.

Restrictive Cultural Food Practices

It has been known for over forty years that restricting the total intake of food in mice, without modifying the proportion of the food constituents could halve the incidence of breast cancer, lung cancer and a variety of other spontaneous tumours.

For ethical and practical reasons such experiments are difficult to conduct in human beings and one has to wait for accidental examples where for geographical, religious or cultural reasons, two populations have differed for decades in their dietary habits: for example, there is a great deal to be learned about the effects of special diets from aboriginal tribes and from primitive communities whose dietary habits differ in certain factors from those obtaining in Western society.

The Kung Bushmen
The Kung Bushmen are a tribe living in North West Botswana, where they are separated from modern

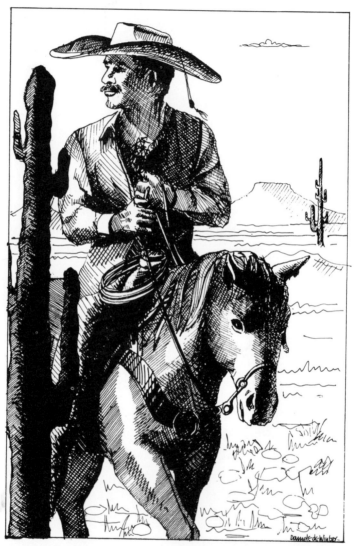

South American Gauchos possess a fine physique because they eat an excess of animal proteins which are excellent body builders.

civilization by a 200 mile wide strip of arid land. As a result, they remain primitive hunter-gatherers and live exclusively on a mixed diet of the fatless meat of the wild buck and the Mungongo nut which is rich in protein and linoleic acid. They have to hunt for their food and having no facilities for storing, have to share. Thus they are not overfed; because engaging as they do in the regular physical exertion of hunting, they remain slim and obesity is almost unknown; being omnivorous there is no malnutrition; having no salt they have a low blood pressure and do not develop strokes; no sugar means that there is little tooth decay or diabetes; their diet being that of fat-free lean meat, cholesterol levels are low and heart disease is virtually unknown. In fact the Kung Bushmen enjoy good health, they are excellent survivors, and their numbers are stable.

Rangers, Gauchos and Masai Warriors

Australian Rangers, South American Gauchos and the African Masai tribesmen eat a *minimum* of 300g (10oz.) of meat per day.

They all possess very fine physiques (as do the milk-drinking Sikhs) because animal proteins are high class proteins which are excellent body builders. Vegetable proteins, on the other hand, are inferior as body builders; hence the much slighter stature of the rice-eating Bengalis.

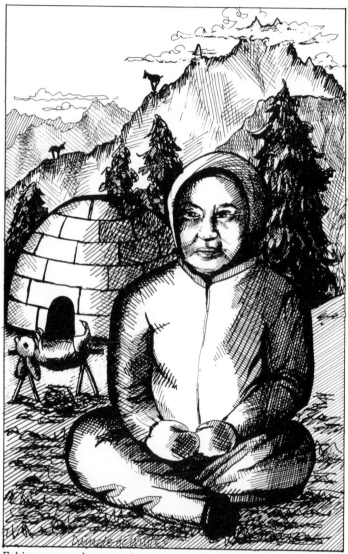

Eskimos are robust carnivorous people who are healthy but age prematurely, possibly as a result of a one-sided unbalanced meat diet.

Eskimos

Eskimos are robust, carnivorous people who exist exclusively on meat and eat no refined carbohydrates or salt. Because they lead a life of great activity and engage in vigorous exercise they remain in excellent health. No cancer or heart disease was found among the indigenous Eskimos in Labrador until they came to live in white man's settlements and adopted the white man's diet and other living habits.

However, Eskimos age prematurely and rapidly, starting at 50; this may possibly be related to their one-sided unbalanced meat diet.

The Hunzas

Another simple community, the Hunzas in India, who are noted for their robust health *and* longevity eat, by way of contrast, a well-balanced mainly vegetarian diet with little protein, fat and sugar.

The Hos Tribe

Members of the Hos tribe in the Province of Bihar in India go even further; they live on a fatless diet. All their food is boiled, they drink no milk and eat no meat so that their fat intake is 2.4g per day — 2% of their total energy intake (compared to 40% fat intake in the West). Not surprisingly, they are in excellent health, as fat is the least necesary item in a healthy diet.

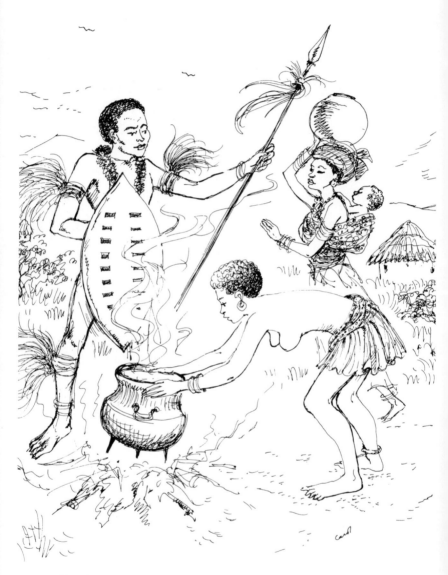

Rural Zulus eat about 8g of sugar a day and diabetes among them is unknown

The Zulus

The ill-effects of sugar are demonstrated by the difference in diet between Zulus living in rural areas and those who are town-dwelling. Most rural Zulus eat about 8g of sugar a day and diabetes among them is virtually unknown, whereas urban Zulus consume up to 100g of sugar a day and their incidence of diabetes is similar to that in the West, where the disease affects one person in seven. Since it increases by 6% every year it follows that the total incidence of diabetes in the West will double every 17 years.

Bantus and Yemen Jews

Rural Bantus who consume 6g of sugar a day show a very low incidence of heart disease when compared with urban Bantus who eat 60g of sugar a day and frequently suffer from heart disease. Jews living in the Yemen average about 6g of sugar a day and rarely suffer from heart disease, but once repatriated to Israel their sugar consumption increases to over 60g and the incidence of heart disease rises correspondingly.

There is a direct link between sugar consumption and the incidence of heart disease conditional on the balance of two fatty substances in the blood: the high and low-density lipo-proteins. The high-density type carries cholesterol into the cell and is protective whereas the low-density lipo-proteins act as a vehicle

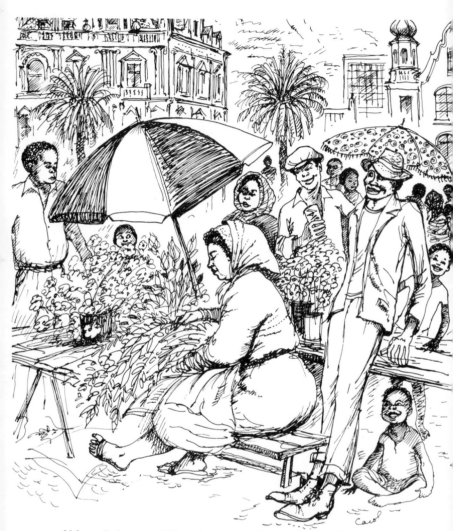

Urban Zulus eat 100g of sugar a day and their incidence of diabetes is similar to that in the West where it affects one person in seven.

Rural Bantus who eat no sugar have practically no heart disease whereas the incidence in Urban Bantus is widespread.

for transporting the blood cholesterol to extracellular tissue, such as the lining of blood vessels. Since sugar intake reduces the level of the protective high-density lipo-proteins it allows the low-density type to pre-dominate, and thereby permits cholesterol to be more readily deposited on the walls of blood vessels, leading to atherosclerosis, hypertension and heart disease.

Anaemia in Bantus

Bantus do not suffer from anaemia because they cook their maize in iron pots and some of the iron always rubs off during cooking and is consumed with the food. Furthermore their favourite drink is a beer very rich in iron.

Bantus apart, anaemia is very widespread in the world: only 3% of Western men, but 25% of Western women are affected. In the third world it affects 40% of women. The total number of women suffering from anaemia worldwide is estimated to be 500 million. In adults, anaemia generally leads only to lack of energy and quick fatigue, but in an expectant mother the disease, endemic in the developing countries, will cause a sixfold increase in the incidence of stillbirths and the infants who manage to survive will be retarded and threatened by illness. Yet supplementary iron in tablet form is inexpensive and easy to take; alternatively either a teaspoon of curry powder or a tablespoon of cocoa or of treacle will provide a third of the daily needs.

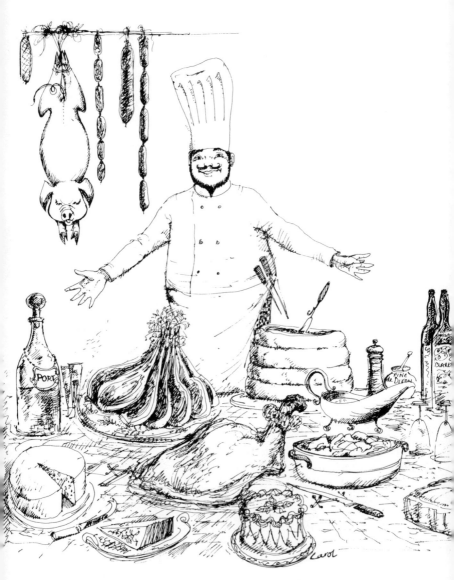

Overfed communities in the affluent West who eat a diet rich in
fat are at much greater risk from heart disease and cancer.

Jewish women of European, Asian and African origin

Different population groups in various parts of the world which have ethnic similarities but different food-styles emphasize the dangers inherent in a fat-rich diet. For instance Jewish women living in New York and Jewish women of European origin but now living in Israel, both eat food that is rich in fat; they both have a significantly higher incidence of cancer and heart disease than Jewish women now living in Israel who originate from Africa and Asia and who prefer food containing little fat.

The serious threat to health from obesity springs from the connection between the hormone level in the blood and degree of obesity on the one hand, and the relationship between a raised hormone level and an increased cancer rate on the other. In the case of menopausal women, it is the obesity which, by increasing the endogenous oestrogen level, is directly responsible for the increased incidence of cancers of the breast, uterus and ovaries.

Seventh Day Adventists and Mormons

Overfed communities in the affluent West who eat a diet rich in fat are much more prone to heart disease and cancer than evangelical sects such as the Seventh Day Adventists or the Mormons who because of their

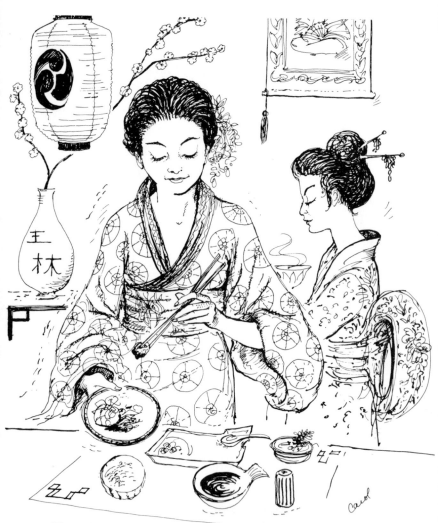

That salt may contribute to high blood pressure is demonstrated in Japan where strokes are the leading cause of death. Since it is difficult to determine in advance who is and who is not sensitive to salt it is a reasonable precaution for everyone to modify the intake.

religion, are abstemious and observe a frugal diet.

Salt The Northern and Southern Japanese

Salt may contribute directly to high blood pressure. Statistically the link is clear and there is a most striking example in Japan. The Southern Japanese consume nearly three teaspoons of salt daily whereas in the Northern agricultural provinces, they consume twice as much — that is six or more teaspoons. As a result Northern Japanese have the highest rate of hypertension in the world which in some villages affects 40% of the population. The incidence of strokes too, (which by the way is the leading cause of death in all Japan) is twice as high in the North than it is in the South.

On the other hand, primitive tribesmen in New Guinea, Malaysia or Uganda eschew salt altogether and there raised blood pressure is virtually unheard of. Thus, since it is difficult to determine in advance who is and who is not sensitive to salt and hypertension, it is a reasonable precaution to modify the intake for everyone.

Vegetarianism

This subject is touched on solely because of its direct effect on wholesome living. The advantages of being a vegetarian lie first in the reduced consumption

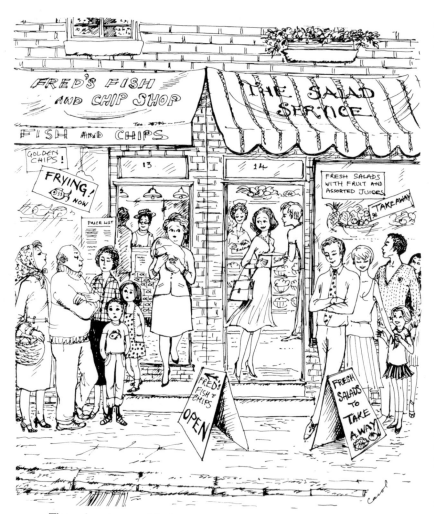

The advantages of being a vegetarian lie first in the reduced consumption of saturated fat and cholesterol contained in fatty meat, and second in the increased intake of dietary fibre, that is roughage, which can be eaten in large amounts in the form of low-calorie and therefore non-fattening vegetables in contrast to the fat-rich and therefore high-calorie fried fish and chips.

of saturated fat and cholesterol which are contained in fatty meat, and second in the increased intake of dietary fibre, that is roughage, eaten in large amounts in the form of vegetables. However the foods *not* eaten, namely: meat, fish and poultry, which are a source of protein, Vitamin B and iron, must be adequately replaced if nutritional deficiencies are to be avoided.

Veganism

This is vegetarianism taken to its logical conclusion. Besides refusing to eat meat, fish and poultry, Vegans also exclude any products of animal origin, including milk, eggs, butter and cheese. Veganism makes it more difficult, though still possible, for all required nutrients to be included in the diet. It is worth recalling that there are many people in the world who live, by necessity, not from choice, on a similarly restricted diet and appear as healthy as most other people.

The Basic Macrobiotic Diet

This diet consists of 50% cooked whole grain such as brown rice, whole wheat or barley, 25% fresh vegetables, 15% beans and the remainder eaten as fish, nuts and fruit. This is a healthy balanced low fat, all-but-vegetarian diet, which can do nothing but good for those sufficiently determined to accept it.

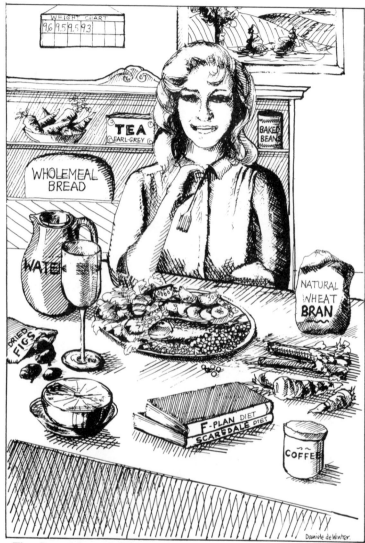

The Scarsdale and F-Plan Diets are well thought out balanced and absolutely safe high-protein, low-carbohydrate and fibre-rich regimes which, if adhered to, will lead to a steady loss of weight.

The Scarsdale and The F-Plan Diets

The principles underlying these two slimming regimes are similar in that to a varying degree they both advocate a mixed, nutritionally well-balanced protein diet with particular emphasis on high-fibre content and severe restriction of all fats and sugar. They are safe diets when used by the healthy. Both will lead to a steady loss of weight only as long as the rules are strictly adhered to.

The Pritkin Diet

This diet is composed of 10% protein, 10% fat and 80% unrefined carbohydrates. Though somewhat drastic, it is a safe diet which, however, disallows much that one most enjoys in the way of everyday culinary pleasures.

It is used in California for the rehabilitation of people suffering from such degenerative illnesses as heart disease and cancer, with good temporary effect.

It should be noted that the basic principles underlying the restrictive Macrobiotic, Scarsdale, F-Plan and Pritkin diets are similar to those advocated in a less extreme, more natural and therefore more effective form throughout this book: *"A stitch in time . . . . .!"*

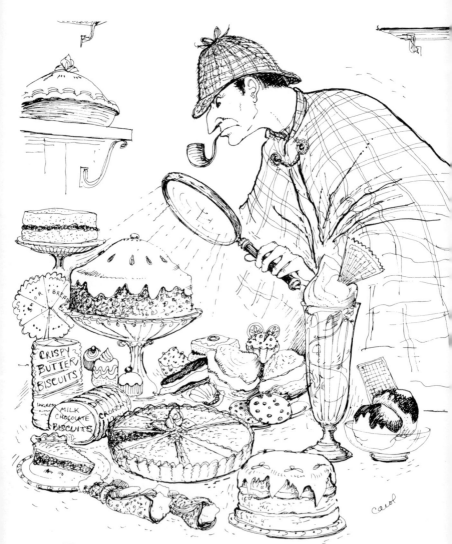

The uniquely unhealthy combination of invisible fats and refined sugar is contained in cakes, puddings and biscuits. If eaten regularly their high content in empty calories will inevitably lead to a gain in weight.

Dietary myths and the truth

There probably exist more preconceived ideas, superstitions and prejudices on the subject of food than on any other topic of corresponding popularity. Some of these misconceptions have been handed down from generation to generation, others have been misleadingly publicised by the media and even more have arisen as a result of unscrupulously slanted and profit-motivated commercial advertising. The following paragraphs attempt to explode some of the myths, to correct some of the misapprehensions and to fill in some of the deliberate omissions.

Biscuits It is never stated in advertisements promoting special brands of biscuits that they contain the uniquely unhealthy combination of pure fat and refined sugar! Nor is it stressed that because of this they are totally lacking in nutriment and that if eaten regularly their high content of empty calories must inevitably lead to a gain in weight.

Cakes Similarly, it is an intentionally misleading psychological manipulation for commercial ends that links home-making with baking a cake. What is not

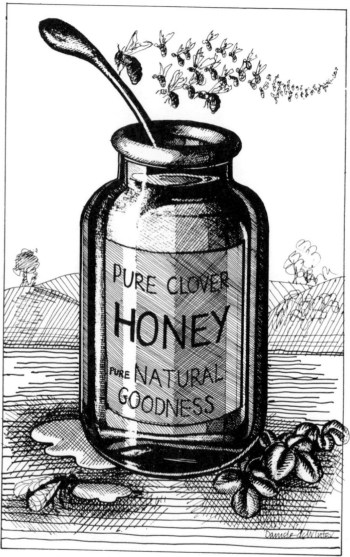

Honey is nothing more than refined sugar and therefore serves no useful medical purpose.

mentioned is that during cake-baking the nutritious flour which contains 10% of protein is corrupted, first by sugar which contains no protein, and then further diluted by fat, which also contains no protein. This means that the resulting flour-confectionery is much less nutritious than the original flour and may even be harmful by contributing to obesity.

Honey There is an aura of romance and magic surrounding the beneficial effects of honey. Contrary to most honey-lovers' deeply held conviction, honey is nothing more than refined sugar, which may well please the palate but which serves no other useful medical purpose.

Similarly the assumed magical effect of bees' Royal Jelly, alleged to have a rejuvenating effect, is totally false. Admittedly the Royal Jelly transforms worker bees into queen bees but, considering the size of a bee, the relative dose for a human being would have to be 20 tons and that presupposes that one would wish to be transformed into a queen bee!

Yoghurt This is another food with alleged "magical" properties! It should be explained that the intestine is the natural home of micro-organisms which help in the formation of stools; these putrefactive bacteria, according to ancient myth, were alleged to have a shortening effect on one's lifespan.

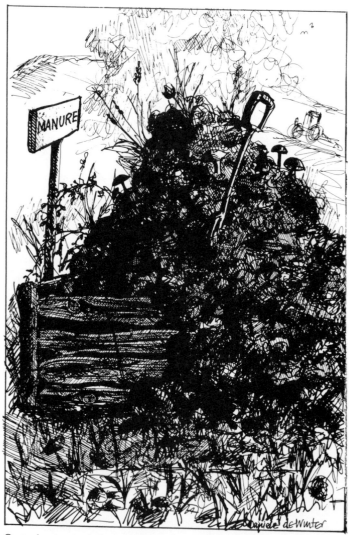

Organic manure from animal droppings contains the identical active agents namely potash, phosphates and sulphate of ammonia which are found in artificial, inorganic, chemically produced fertilizers.

Because yoghurt contains different, that is souring, bacteria, it was thought that these would neutralize the stool's own "life-shortening" bacteria and in this way prolong life. A good story, but totally untrue, as myths usually are!

Sea-salt A great deal has been claimed about the superiority of sea-salt over ordinary cooking salt; it contains a small amount of iodine, but in a non-landlocked country there is an ample supply of iodine in the normal food anyway. Otherwise sea-salt only contains impurities of sea-water and is therefore medically valueless and, at the same time, much more expensive.

Vitamin E This Vitamin is available in adequate amounts in most natural foods and therefore no supplement is necessary. Vitamin E has been dubbed the Vitamin "in search of a disease" because it has no known medicinal value in adults.

Organically Grown Food

Organic manure and fertilisers in the form of animal droppings, compost, blood meal, hoof and horn meal, as used by old-fashioned gardeners, can be utilized by nature only after these substances have been broken down into their basic chemical constituents, namely potash, phosphate and sulphate of ammonia. These

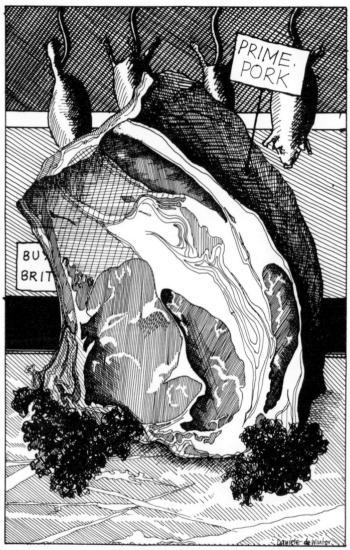

Meat as sold on the slab by the butcher contains 50% fat, whereas lean meat only has 5% fat with 20% protein and 75% water.

three substances are in fact the main ingredients of the so-called inorganic or chemical fertilisers. The only conceivable advantage of natural, organic manure and compost is that they loosen up the soil and release their chemical constituents gradually.

Meat It is not correct, as claimed by many butchers, that the most tender portions of meat are the fat cuts. Whereas lean meat contains only 5% fat with 20% protein and 75% water, meat as sold on the slab has 50% of fat. Neither is it true that the white meat of poultry is more nutritious than red meat. What *is* true is that poultry, being leaner, contains less fat and cholesterol, and is therefore healthier. Although fat meat is not quickly digested because the fat delays emptying of the stomach and thus increases the "full-up" feeling, a healthy stomach has no difficulty in digesting fat. Nevertheless all fat should be cut off the meat before cooking and should never be eaten.

Hung Meat What makes meat tough is its indigestible fibrous tissue. Hunted animals produce quantities of lactic acid just prior to death, due to intense muscular activity. This acid gelatinises the fibres and tenderises the meat. Farm animals, slaughtered whilst standing still, give less tender meat, but acids continue to form after death in the muscles and that is why hung meat becomes more tender with time.

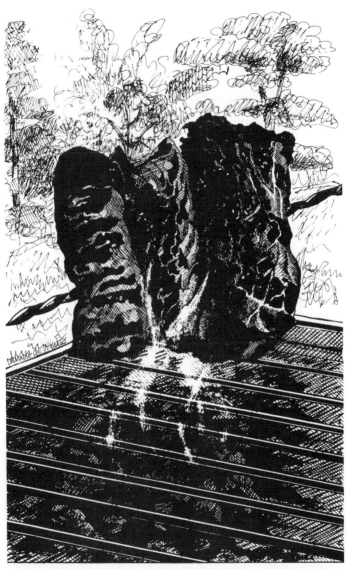

Meat charred black on barbecuing can contain powerful carcinogens in the areas exposed to very high temperatures.

Free-range Meat There is some controversy about the food-value of free-range meat compared with stall-fed meat. Both are equally nutritious but feed-lots produce fat meat whereas free-range meat is much leaner; in fact farmers already have the knowledge (but are reluctant to use it because it would be commercially less profitable), to raise cow-breeds with low-fat milk and low-fat meat. The priceless benefits for the public that would accrue from these specially bred fatless cattle-species would include sausages, hamburgers and hot dogs with lean meat, and dairy products with low saturated-fat content.

Barbecues Charcoal-grilling of steaks at barbecues, until the outside of the meat is charred black, can produce powerful carcinogens in the areas subjected to the very high temperatures and should be avoided because these carcinogens are known to produce cancer in animals. However, good cooks do not usually pyrolyse much of the food they are cooking, although they may caramelize it. In normal circumstances the temperatures involved in barbecue cooking rarely exceed 200°C, which is quite safe.

Meat and Health Better health is not, as frequently stated, the result of greater meat consumption. It is due to a balanced diet consisting of proteins, minerals and vitamins.

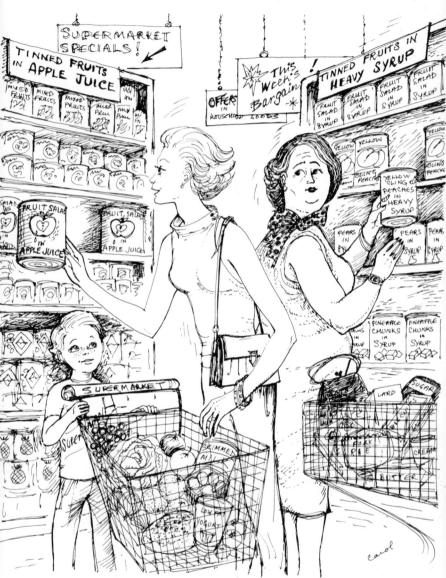

Shop sensibly with an eye on products low in fat and sugar.

Eating more meat puts an extra burden on the kidneys. Even though healthy kidneys are perfectly able to excrete the resulting greatly increased amounts of nitrogen, there are three potentially harmful side-effects that such a high meat consumption entails:

1. The toxic by-products of increased protein metabolism, such as uric acid, urea and ammonia, when present in excess, can contribute to arthritis and other illnesses.

2. If all the protein eaten by the high meat consumption is not used up for energy, the excess will be stored as fat.

3. Since all animal protein is rich in cholesterol, increased meat consumption will be harmful to people with a predisposition to heart disease and high blood pressure. Since we cannot tell in advance who is and who is not so predisposed, it is best to restrict the intake of meat at all times.

Slimming Cures It is understandable that in the search for the quickest slimming "cures" even more intelligent people become gullible and put their faith in all kinds of magical diets. Some, for example, believe that as long as they start each meal with a grapefruit, they can eat as much as they wish during the subsequent meal without gaining weight! Of course, this is nonsense.

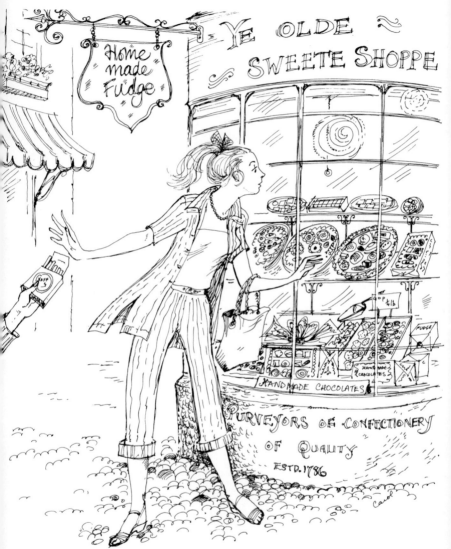

Giving up smoking creates a craving for sweets and it may take the body six months to re-adjust to the absence of the noxious though weight-reducing effects of cigarettes.

Another misconception is that a limit of two meals a day will ensure a loss of weight. The truth is that it is the *calorie content* of the food which is the determining factor. Provided that the total eaten is the same, *five small meals* are more slimming than two large ones, because at each meal some of the consumed energy is dissipated in the form of heat.

Slimming is helped by eating slowly and masticating well. This causes more saliva to be formed which helps to fill the stomach; by eating slowly one might therefore well eat less.

There are three main reasons why cigarettes help to keep smokers slim. Firstly smoking depresses appetite and a smoker therefore tends to eat less; then it speeds up digestion so there is less time for fat to be absorbed and stored. Finally, each cigarette releases sugar into the bloodstream, so there is no desire for sugar and other sweet foods.

Conversely, once smoking is given up, all these weight-reducing factors are reversed: the appetite increases, digestion is slowed down, and occasionally there is an irresistible craving for sugar. The result is a rapid weight-gain in the initial period after giving up the habit and it sometimes takes the body at least six months to re-adjust to the absence of the noxious, though weight-reducing, effects of cigarettes.

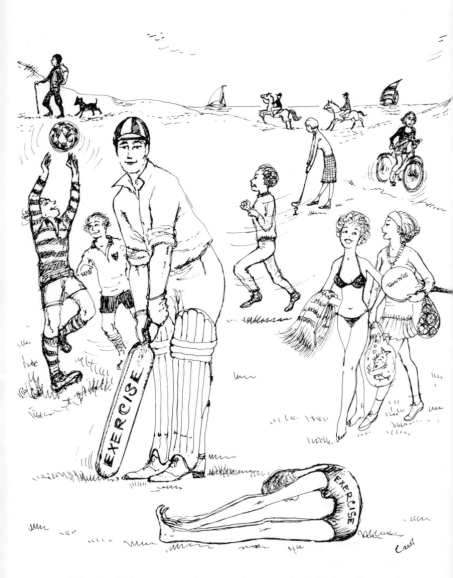

The healthiest person is one who spends a lifetime in regular vigorous outdoor exercise.

Physical Exercise

There is ample evidence that lack of exercise contributes to the risk of atherosclerosis (hardening of the arteries), heart disease, hypertension (high blood pressure), strokes, obesity, diabetes and, last but not least, constipation.

One of the best ways of eliminating poisonous waste products which have accumulated in the body is regular exercise. This will restore the proper balance of the many essential constituents in the blood, and additionally, tends to release pent-up emotions and relieve mental stress.

The main purpose of exercise is to increase the efficiency of the heart and lungs, and it should be taken regularly, preferably for a period of 30-60 minutes at least five times per week — throughout an entire lifetime.

It is immaterial how exercise is taken; whether in the form of the "daily dozen" or taking a long, brisk walk instead of driving the car or taking a bus; running upstairs two at a time rather than taking the lift; cycling long distances or energetically digging the

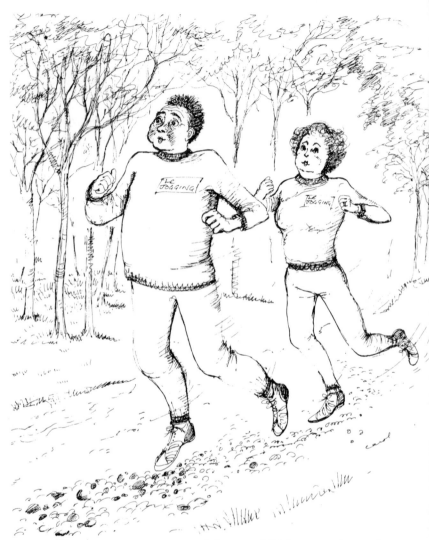

There are many unsuccessful overweight joggers who, unless they cut down on fats, sugar and alcohol, will always remain fat because even in extended exercises little of the massive energy contained in the food can be used up.

garden. All these physical exertions in fit people should be gradually increased both in duration and vigour until a state of pronounced breathlessness and a marked increase in pulse rate is experienced at least once every day. However, even in extended vigorous exercises little of the massive energy contained in the dietary fat or sugar is used up; that is why there are so many unsuccessful overweight joggers who, unless they cut down on fats, sugar and alcohol, will always remain fat.

For the energetic business executive exercise is also the only reliable method of protection from the stresses of his life, particularly as these usually include heavy smoking and hard drinking as well as over-eating. In such cases, systematic physical exercise may well assume a life-saving role, when otherwise a heart attack, or a stroke may be only a matter of time.

There is conclusive evidence that people fortunate enough to be able to engage in regular sporting activities are, as a result of the healthy exercise, usually in excellent mental and physical condition. They are generally relaxed and sleep well; they worry less and they have no desire to over-eat or smoke, neither do they crave alcohol. Not only is their blood pressure normal, their pulse rate is slow at rest, and even more important, it increases only slightly on exertion.

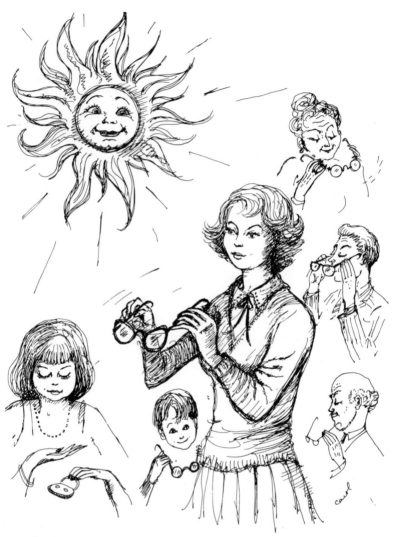

Outdoor activities afford the added bonus of unfiltered sunlight entering the eyes through the pupils, which is essential for optimal body conditions. Since the glass used for ordinary spectacles and contact lenses filters out ultraviolet light, these should be removed from time to time.

Outdoor sports afford the added bonus of natural unfiltered sunlight which is essential for optimal body condition. Natural light affects the body's hormone system after entering the eyes through the pupils. This results in a general sense of well-being as well as an increase in efficiency and a decrease in fatigue and explains why natural sunlight has such a very significant association with a person's mood. Since the glass used for ordinary spectacles and contact lenses filters out ultraviolet light, these should be removed from time to time, or they should be made of special material which does not shield out ultraviolet light.

To summarize: Physical exercise is better by far than any known drug or medicine because it cures more diseases, solves more problems and relieves more stress than any other single agent. In particular, by burning excess blood-fat for fuel and cleaning the arteries of their fatty deposits, it minimizes the risk of atherosclerosis and prevents high blood pressure, strokes, heart disease, obesity, diabetes and gallstones — the disastrous consequences of stress, sloth and gluttony. One further important advantage of exercise is its stimulating effect on intestinal peristalsis which helps to prevent constipation and with it a host of complicating illnesses.

In short, the healthiest person is one who spends a lifetime in regular vigorous outdoor exercise. The best

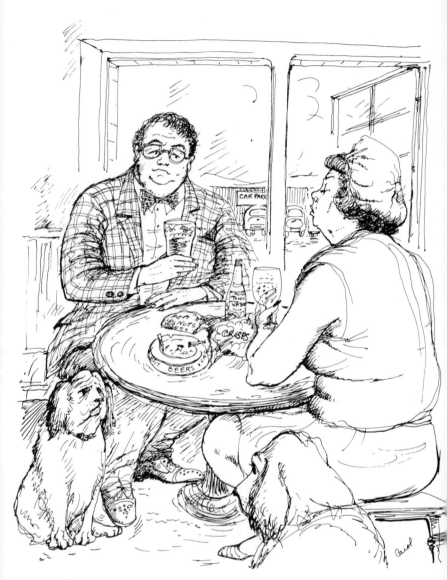

Basically a sedentary person is sick and those who do not find time for exercise will later have to find time for sickness.

exercises are those demanding endurance. Basically, a sedentary person is sick and those who do not find time for exercise will later *have* to find time for sickness.

Questions on Exercise

(Any answer in the affirmative is favourable)

Do you like exercise

Do you go for brisk walks

Do you climb stairs

Do you do gymnastics

Do you engage in sport

Do you feel the need for exercise

Do you like to get breathless

Is your weight steady

Have you lost weight

Are you determined not to gain weight

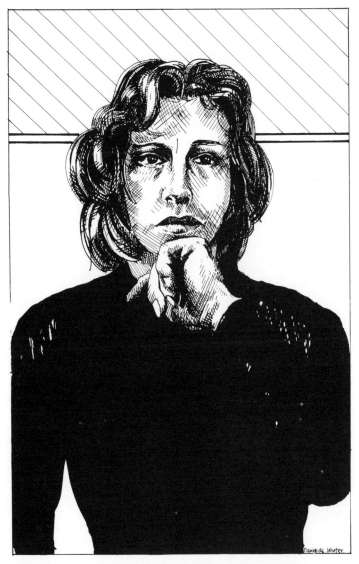

Negative emotions such as fear, anxiety, anger and jealousy can be as harmful to health as dietary excesses.

Emotional Stress

Emotional stress is a condition known to contribute to heart disease, high blood pressure, strokes and cancer.

A human being is not merely a chemical factory or a primitive biological creature but an entity, comprising body, mind and spirit. It is the harmonious inter-relationship of these three components which determines one's state of well-being.

Stress has a debilitating effect on the body's immune system; though it is not the actual cause of the illness, it may be the determinant factor which swings the balance in a borderline condition. This is why certain illnesses cannot be explained in purely physical terms and why other factors such as anxiety, insecurity, emotional tension and stress play such an important part in their causation. Anxious people take much more out of themselves and thus become vulnerable to ill health. Nor is it unusual that the onset of illnesses such as cancer, a stroke or a coronary heart attack can be related to an emotional

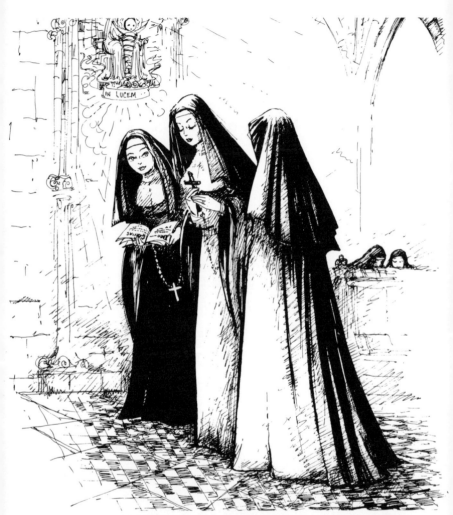

The relaxation technique of "mindless prayer", which involves repeating a phrase or prayer in tranquil surroundings and which has been in use throughout the world for thousands of years, can have a beneficial effect on patients at risk from heart disease or high blood pressure, by reducing excessive amounts of the hormone Noradrenalin, which is produced under stress.

upset. In fact it is possible to predict by taking personality into account, which individuals in a group are more prone eventually to contract one or other of these illnesses. Unless helped by counselling and meditation the troubled mind in such cases may continue to transmit its harmful messages to the body thereby altering its normal chemistry.

In summary, because negative emotions such as fear, anxiety, anger and jealousy can be as harmful to health as dietary excesses, one must deliberately eliminate them by voicing one's feelings freely to avoid the build up of nervous tension which may lead to mental stress. For many, prayer and contemplation may be very effective by contributing to a more relaxed attitude of mind, but because the beneficial effects of meditation are still considered scientifically unproven, there are few reputable centres where this ancient method of mental relaxation is accepted as orthodox treatment. Other relaxation techniques which involve repeating a phrase or a prayer in comfortable quiet surroundings have been in use throughout the world for thousands of years and their beneficial effect, particularly in patients at risk from heart disease or high blood pressure, is irrefutable. This technique of "mindless" prayer is thought to reduce excessive amounts of the hormone Noradrenaline which is produced under stress.

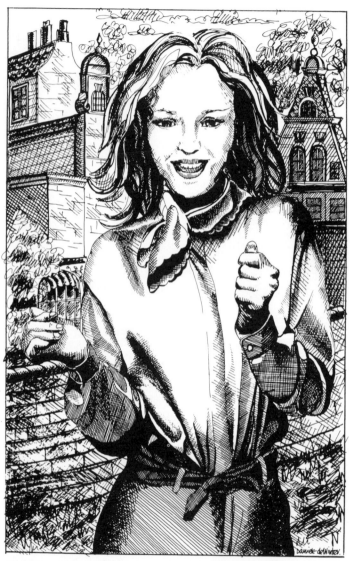

Positive emotions such as love, joy and contentment avoid the build-up of tension which is known to lead to emotional stress.

Questions on Emotional Stress
(Any answer in the affirmative is favourable)

Are you calm and confident

Do you sleep well

Do you find time to contemplate

Do you meditate

Have you a desire to help others

Do you have someone to love

Do you have someone you can lean on

Are you glad to be alive

Are you able to express your emotions

Does your work satisfy you

(Any answer in the affirmative is unfavourable)

Are you nervous and insecure

Do you worry about things

Are you particularly afraid of cancer

Are you easily angry

Are you inclined to bottle up your feelings

Do you tend to be jealous

Do you feel lonely

Do you feel fed up

Do you easily harbour a grudge

Are you often depressed

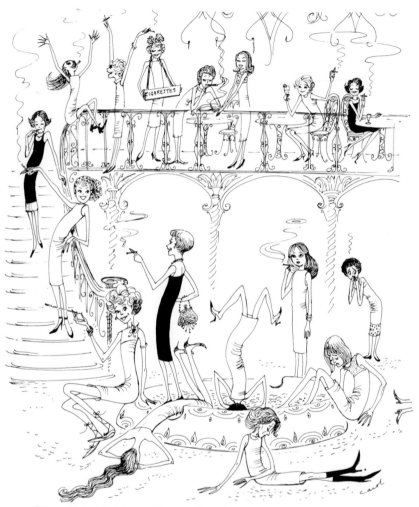

There is irrefutable evidence that cigarette smoking is the main cause of heart disease, high blood pressure, strokes, lung cancer, chronic bronchitis, emphysema and bladder cancer. In women lung cancer death-rates have trebled in the last 15 years as a result of the increased number of women who have taken up smoking.

Cigarettes

There is ample and conclusive evidence of the disastrous effects of cigarette smoking. It contributes to heart disease, arteriosclerosis, high blood pressure, strokes, lung cancer, chronic bronchitis, emphysema and bladder cancer.

The three noxious agents of tobacco responsible for the damage to health are:

1. **Tar,** which causes lung cancer. It also causes the deadly chronic bronchitis and bladder cancer. By destroying the protein which protects the elastic tissues lining the lung, it is an important cause of emphysema, a condition in which the loss of tissue elasticity makes exhalation progressively more difficult.

2. **Nicotine** which produces two contrasting effects. First, it creates an anaesthetic-like state of mental tranquility and relaxation. Second, by releasing adrenalin and sugar, it makes the smoker feel alert and ready to cope with any emergency.
   These two states together produce yet a third state, that of a continuous craving for cigarettes and total addiction.

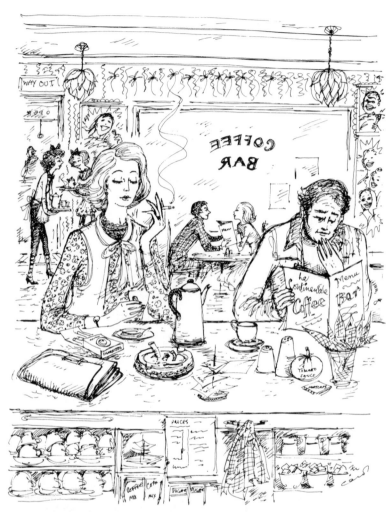

It is the carbon monoxide concentration in the cigarettes which causes the clogging-up of arteries by raising the blood level of the lipid carrying the cholesterol to the blood vessel walls as a result of which the blood vessels become progressively blocked. This risk is increased in women over 35 taking "the pill" who are also regular smokers.

3. **Carbon monoxide** concentration (higher in cigarettes *with* filters) which causes hardening of the arteries by raising the blood level of the low density faction lipid carrying cholesterol. This faction gets deposited in the walls of damaged blood vessels which ultimately become blocked, thus cutting off the blood supply and causing the death of parts of vital organs, such as the heart (coronary thrombosis), the brain (stroke), or the foot (gangrene).

Since contraceptive pills increase the clotting tendency of the blood, women over the age of 35 taking the pill who are also regular smokers run a much higher risk of cerebral thrombosis (a stroke) and should cease smoking.

Questions on Cigarettes

(Any answer in the affirmative is unfavourable)

Do you smoke 10 or more cigarettes a day

Have you smoked for 10 or more years

Do you smoke most of each cigarette

Do you inhale

Have you given up smoking and resumed

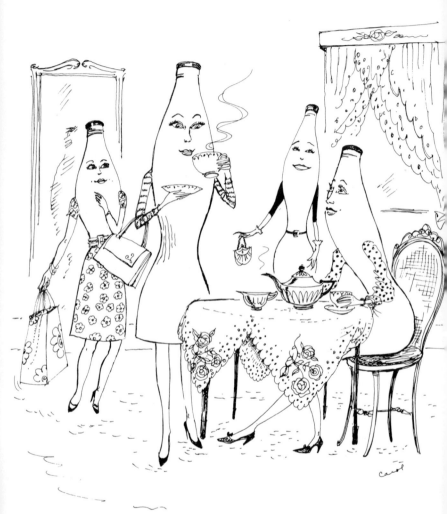

Whole milk presents great disadvantages over skimmed milk. Whereas the protein, carbohydrate and vitamin content is identical in both, there are 200 calories in one pint of skimmed milk but 375, nearly double, the calories in one pint of whole milk which is exclusively due to the presence of fat, one of the least necessary substances in a healthy diet.

Breast and Cervix

The breast appears particularly prone to react to excessive milk-fat consumption, in that breast cancer mortality correlates more strongly with the consumption of milk-fat than with other types of fat. Whole milk is a high-calorie food which presents grave disadvantages over skimmed milk. Whereas the protein, vitamin and carbohydrate content is identical in both, the fat content of skimmed milk is one twentieth that of whole milk which means that there are only 200 calories in one pint of skimmed milk, but 375 nearly *double* the calories in one pint of whole milk. This high-calorie content of whole milk is exclusively due to the presence of fat, a substance which, though pleasing to the palate, can be harmful to health.

Another factor affecting the breast is childbirth, in that the development of breast cancer in child-bearing women becomes progressively less likely as the age of the first pregnancy decreases. The earlier the first pregnancy, the less likely is the woman to suffer from

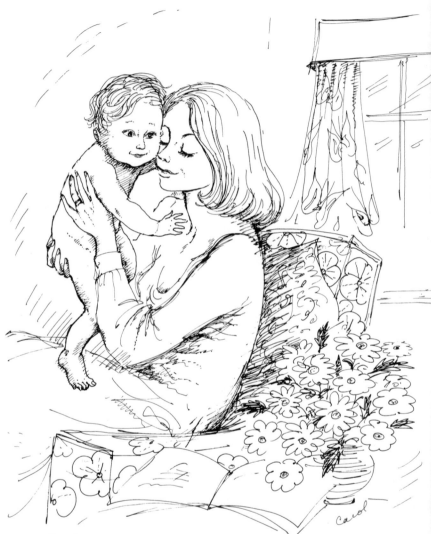

Development of breast cancer in child-bearing women becomes progressively less likely as the age of the first pregnancy decreases. Altogether pregnancies appear to have a protective effect with cancers of the breast, ovary and body of the uterus.

breast cancer. This may be due to the effect of the first stimulus to lactation. This diminished risk is re-inforced by a late onset of menstruation at puberty, particularly when this was due to under-nutrition: another example of the protective effect on health of dietary restriction. On the other hand over-nutrition and the resulting obesity increases the risk of both breast and uterine cancer.

The other frequent form of cancer in women is cancer of the cervix, a form of cancer that spares nuns and virgins. It is obviously related to the sexual act and is commonest in prostitutes. This risk can be greatly reduced by:

1. Postponing the practice of regular intercourse until well beyond the 'teens.
2. By using a barrier contraceptive
3. By having a single partner
4. By making one's partner, especially if uncircumcised, wash thoroughly behind the foreskin before intercourse.
5. By having a hot bath immediately after intercourse, with scrupulous cleansing of the vagina. This is an additional simple measure of immense protective value.

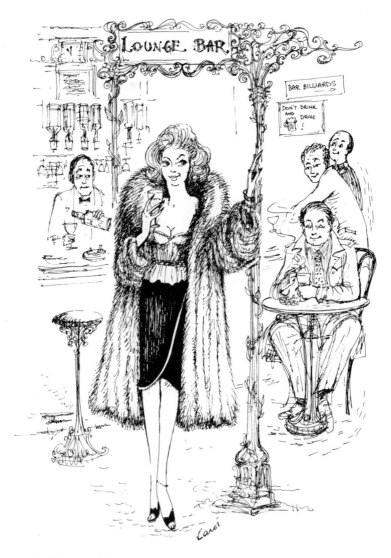

Avoidance of the sexual act would probably eliminate cancer of the cervix which is a form of cancer that spares virgins but is commonest in prostitutes.

Questions on Breast and Cervix:

(Any answer in the affirmative is unfavourable)

Do your breasts get lumpy

Is there breast cancer in the family

Are you childless

First child after aged 30

Breast feeding unsuccessful

(Any answer in the affirmative is favourable)

Did you start sex after 19

Do your partners wash before sex

Do you wash after sex

Do you avoid sex during a period

Do you use a barrier contraceptive

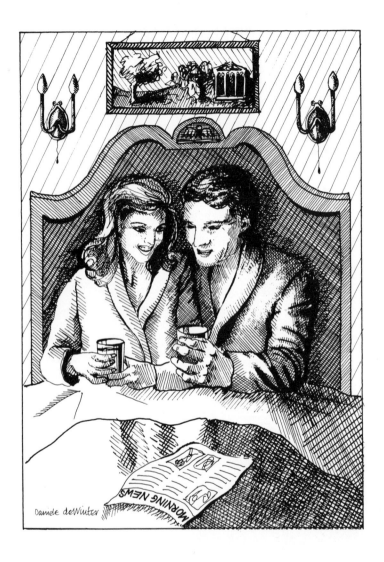

Before getting out of bed one should sit up and drink 2 glasses of water or, if preferred, 3 cups of unsugared weak tea. A total of about 4 pints of water should be drunk each day.

114

A daily routine
to keep one's arteries young

Ideally one should plan to wake up at least 15 minutes before actually having to get up, to give the awakening mind time for serene contemplation as it proceeds to full wakefullness. This should be a smooth and gentle process which can be aided by soothing music but *not* by stressful radio-news.

During this extra lie in, cat-like stretching movements of limbs and spine will loosen the joints after a night of immobility. Before getting out of bed one should sit up and slowly sip 2 glasses of water to help initiate a reflex-peristaltic wave through the intestines to expedite a regular early morning bowel action. Since about 65% of the body is composed of water it is important to replenish the body's water reservoir by drinking about 4 pints of water each day. It should always be drunk slowly while seated, not when standing up.

On rising from bed some simple gymnastic exercises will give further help to the muscles and joints that may have stiffened up overnight. These physical exercises should be followed by breathing

115

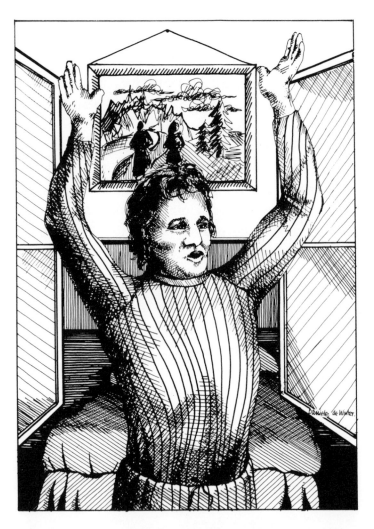

A dozen deep rhythmical inspirations through the nose and expirations every morning and whenever convenient throughout the day will expand to the full the otherwise unused lowermost parts of the lungs and provide additional oxygen without any increased effort by the heart.

exercises consisting of a dozen deep rhythmical inspirations and expirations which will expand the lungs to the full. One should always breathe in through the nose but one may breathe out through either the nose or the mouth. Such breathing exercises should be repeated whenever convenient about every 4 hours throughout the day.

After exercising, one should proceed to the bathroom for a shower and a brisk rub down. Dental hygiene forms a most important part of health care, so the teeth should be thoroughly brushed, (not forgetting to massage the gums) and this process should be repeated after each meal.

As regards clothing one should remember that synthetic fibre like nylon is non-porous and does not allow the skin to breathe, so one should try to wear natural fibre such as cotton, wool or silk next to the skin. It is also important to avoid all constricting garments such as form-fitting jeans. It is better not to wear tight shoes and the heels should be neither too high nor too low, but just comfortable.

Allow at least half an hour for a leisurely breakfast and do not forget to brush your teeth again afterwards.

This very relaxed start, which is very important because it will set one up for the rest of the day, should be compared with the more usual, frenetic

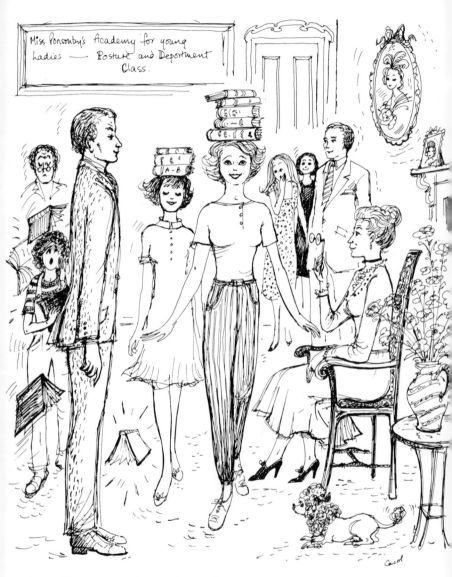

Always try to sit, stand or walk erect, thereby preventing painful aches and pains in the neck or back in later years.

routine practiced in the "civilized"West, where a lightning catapult out of bed is followed by a quick dash to the bathroom, a hurried breakfast and a mad rush out of the house to the garage or to catch a train or bus.

Small wonder, then, after repeating this at least 300 times a year for 35 years, that many will have developed a high blood pressure and will eventually suffer a stroke, which after heart disease and cancer, is the third commonest cause of death.

The type of breakfast to be taken is a matter for individual preference but as a general guide: sugar, butter, cream, whole-milk products, fried eggs, fried bacon and white bread should be restricted whereas crude bran, wholemeal bread and fruit should always be included. It is not generally appreciated how very important it is to masticate well at all times.

It is also important to be always aware of one's posture and to try, consciously, to sit, stand or walk erect. This means upright, with the shoulders well back, the neck straight and the head held high. In this stance the head and the beck becomes a natural extension of the spine and this will prevent many of the painful ailments of the neck, shoulders, arms, back and legs in later life.

Instead of using transport all the way to work, at

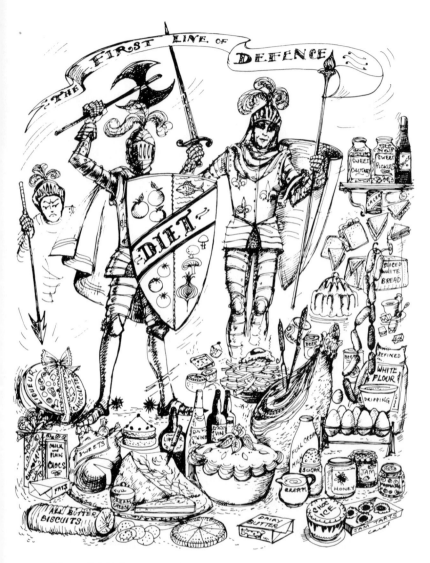

Since 'Diet' forms the first line of defence in the fight against degenerative illness, with fats, sugar and alcohol heading the list of restricted items, modest meals are obligatory on weekdays.

least part of the way should be covered on foot at a fairly brisk pace. This should include all stairs which should be welcomed as an ideal opportunity for sudden physical exertion. For those not going out to work, a vigorous morning walk or cycle ride is imperative before settling down to work at home and if this is of a sedentary nature then the morning's physical activities become absolutely mandatory.

During week-ends, when staying at home, select the sport compatible with age, physical capacity and mental attitude and one should never forget that walking is marvellous as a recreation.

Half-way through a working morning, perhaps during the coffee break, at least 10 minutes should be spent in positive thinking: that is, in serene contemplation, which will re-charge the wearying mind. Before resuming work one should remember deep-breathing exercises and some simple gymnastic movements to relax the muscles and the joints of the spine. This will allow one to resume work refreshed and with renewed zest until lunch time.

A modest lunch is preferable, to be followed by a short brisk walk. During the subsequent rest period use the time for another session of serene contemplation followed by rhythmical deep breathing and light gymnastic movements.

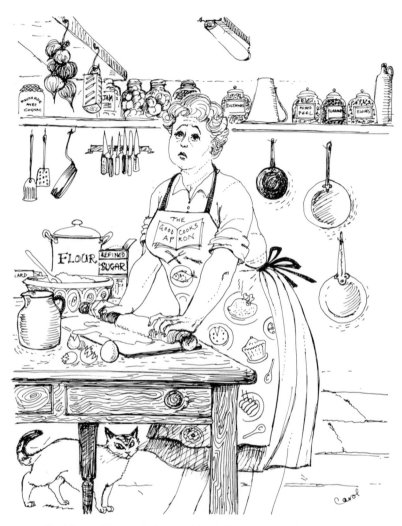

Cooking with much fat and lots of sugar, that is, eating heavy meals, as well as drinking a great deal of alcohol, will lead to obesity and thus to degenerative diseases; restraint at meal times as regards both food and drink is the best insurance against ill-health.

Lunch is a matter of personal preference. Several small meals a day are better than one or two large ones. Yet again: sugar, butter, cream, whole-milk, cheeses, alcohol, fat meat, fried food, ice-creams, cakes and white bread are on the "restricted items list", whilst wholemeal bread, baked or boiled potatoes, vegetables, fruit, fish and poultry are permitted.

Again, part of the homeward journey should be covered on foot. On arrival at home one should ensure a period of light-hearted conversation and relaxation before the evening meal. The art of laughing and of being cheerful should be cultivated at this and all other times, and anger and contention should be avoided. If possible one's philosophy should always be: "Accept with grace what cannot be changed and try to be content with what you have".

Large dinners should be reserved for the odd festive occasion when there is something to celebrate. A heavy meal at night interferes with sound sleep; in any case every large meal enhances the risk of obesity particularly when the food eaten is rich in sugar, fats and alcohol. The diet should always be balanced with the main emphasis being on proteins and roughage, that is on food rich in dietary fibre such as bran, wholemeal flour products, vegetables and fruit. In fact, roughage should proportionally form the largest single

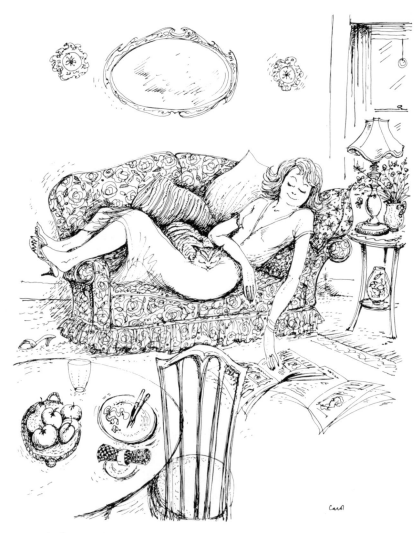

A "cat-nap" in the middle of the day is an important habit to cultivate because a brief period with feet up, eyes closed and complete relaxation will have a re-vitalizing effect for the rest of the day.

item in every meal and this important rule should be always adhered to.

And so to bed. A bedroom should be cool, unheated and airy. One should refrain from taking stimulants such as strong tea, coffee or alcohol after 5pm. To avoid a "bad back", the mattress should be very firm, if not hard, as this promotes sound dreamless sleep and increases the likelihood of waking well rested and in a happy frame of mind.

Whereas 10 hours of sleep are permissible at the age of 20, with advancing years there is a gradually decreasing need for sleep and it is advisable to reduce the time spent in bed. Fit people need only 6-7 hours of sleep.

Conversely, from 20 years and on, it is really important to interrupt one's activities in the middle of the day for a brief rest-period with the feet up, eyes closed and complete mental relaxation. This "cat-nap" is an invaluable asset and very important to cultivate. A 10 minutes rest at the age of 30 should be gradually increased to roughly 20 minutes at the age of 60.

Since natural unfiltered light is essential for optimal body conditions and ordinary spectacles and contact lenses shield out the ultraviolet rays, glasses or contact lenses should be removed for about ten minutes 2 − 3 times each day.

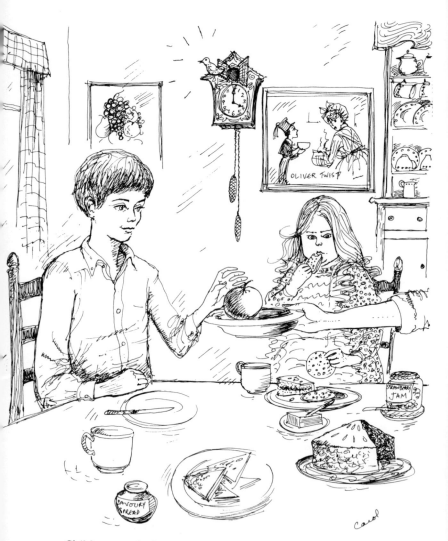

Children taught from early childhood to accept discretion in food, abstemiousness in alcohol and abstention in cigarettes as matters of course, will enjoy an enduring capability for high-quality living throughout their healthy lives.

A Plea to Good Parents

It is undeniable that all adults accustomed to late twentieth-century norms will find the suggested restrictions both irksome and hard to accept.

Yet, when these very same dietary restrictions are introduced in childhood they are readily adopted and quickly become second nature to the child. The earlier one starts the easier it is to continue and the greater will be the subsequent rewards in terms of fitness and well-being.

If, as a result of the good example set by their enlightened parents, today's children could be made to accept from early childhood that discretion in food, abstemiousness in alcohol, abstention in cigarettes, regular physical activity every day of the year and personal responsibility for health and conduct are all matters of course, they would have had bestowed upon them the most precious heritage, namely an enduring capability for high quality living.

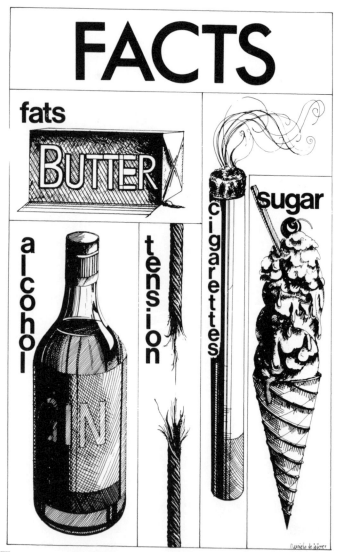

The acronym FACTS stands for Fats, Alcohol, Cigarettes, Tension and Sugar which all are best avoided in the interest of long-term health.

Summary: 10 Health-Precepts

The chances of avoiding premature ageing as well as many of today's disabilities caused by degenerative diseases are immeasurably enhanced by constant observance of 10 health-precepts summed up in the two five-letter acronyms: "FACTS" and "SMART".

The acronym "FACTS" stands for **F**at, **A**lcohol, **C**igarettes, **T**ension and **S**ugar: for long-term good health all five are best avoided, if at all possible.

The acronym "SMART" stands for **S**erenity, **M**oderation, **A**ctivity, **R**oughage and **T**rying. Early adoption of all five is of paramount importance because each one in turn complements the beneficial effects of the others in the quest for lasting health and fulfilment.

Serenity: A high quality of life depends as much on a relaxed mind and a deep faith as on physical well-being.

Moderation: This quite indispensable prerequisite for long term health can be successfully sustained only if based on self-discipline, willpower and motivation.

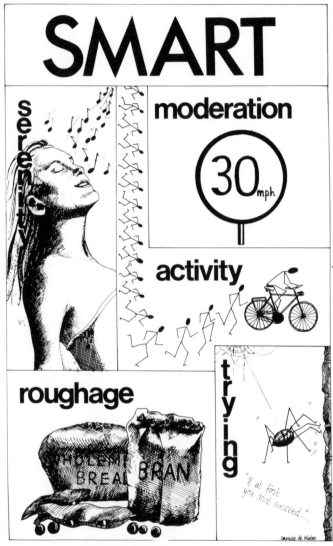

The acronym SMART which stands for Serenity, Moderation, Activity, Roughage and Trying represents the 5 pre-requisites for enduring health.

Activity: Without regular physical exercise the clean, free-flowing, oxygen-rich bloodstream which provides the vital supply of nutrients and oxygen to the tissues, is impeded, leaving the cells malnourished and impurified, that is, laden with waste products which cannot be cleared.

Roughage: Crude fibre-containing foods are easily the most important constituent of one's diet since they absorb toxic substances from the bowel and expedite their excretion by increasing the peristaltic movement of the gut.

Trying: It is only by constant trying, that the control and conquest of one's habitual weaknesses will become second nature.

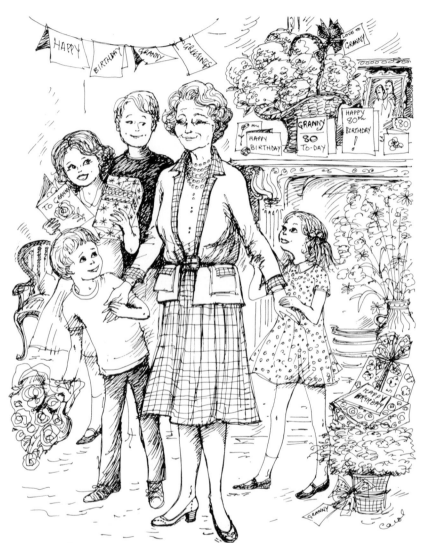

Undimmed vision, unimpaired hearing, undiminished intellect, unspoiled appetite, undisturbed digestion, unrestricted mobility are the essential faculties which, together with peace of mind, are all needed for full enjoyment of life at any age.

Conclusion: A Priceless Bonus

The degree to which life can be enjoyed mainly depends on one's peace of mind and the excellence of such bodily faculties as undimmed vision, unimpaired hearing, undiminished intellect, unspoiled appetite, undisturbed digestion and uncurtailed mobility, to mention but the more important.

With advancing years, even in the absence of obvious ill-health, retention of high quality living will become increasingly more dependent on one's deliberate effort of keeping these faculties intact.

The average person is loth to work for good health — yet good health cannot be achieved without effort, neither can it be bought. There are rules that must be obeyed and the principal one is that dietary habits must be simple, regular, moderate and wholesome. Life's quality hinges far more on the rate at which we let our tissues degenerate than it depends on our actual age. The Bible says that man's allotted span is threescore years and ten but this need not be so. By

133

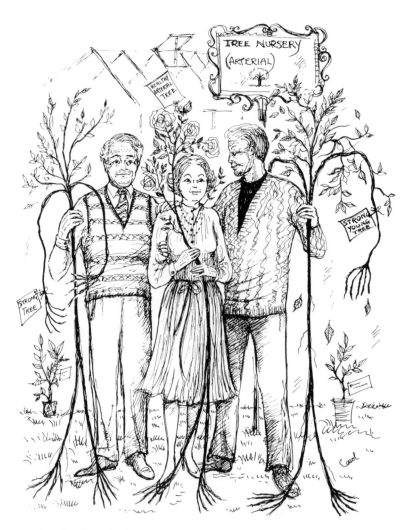

Free-flowing blood in clean, flexible arteries is the best insurance against illness, with a sensible diet as first line of defence and physical activity as a second line. The earlier this philosophy becomes a natural way of life the better the chances of high-quality living beyond eighty.

adhering to the 10 health precepts we can maintain a high-velocity oxygen-rich bloodstream in clear and flexible arteries to keep our body tissues fresh and thereby extend our capability for life's full enjoyment well beyond the allotted span.

The art of living consists of staying young as late as possible. Therefore the earlier self-imposed restraint becomes second nature the better the chances of achieving this.

In other words, earlier adoption of dietary discretion and restraint as a way of life, when coupled with regular and sustained physical activity, will help to prevent premature ageing and with it such illnesses as diabetes, hypertension, strokes, heart disease and cancer, thereby extending the ultimate span of usefulness and personal independence well beyond the eighties.

Appendix:

Degenerative Diseases of Affluence

Obesity: Years ago people had to do hard physical work which demanded heavy exertion for many hours every day. They had to walk many miles to and from their work. Today cars and buses transport us to our jobs and much of the heavy work in factories and at home is mechanised. Small wonder then, that so many people become fat. Body weight can be likened to our income tax liability. If food energy intake (our profit) exceeds output used in physical activity (our business expenses) then the excess will be stored in fat (the excess will be liable to income tax).

Gallstones: Excess cholesterol taken in the diet by eating too much fat, if not eliminated from the body, is stored mainly in the liver. In high concentration, cholesterol forms crystals that eventually accumulate as stones in the gallbladder.

Diabetes: The common but relatively mild forms of adult-onset diabetes are gradually brought on over the years by frequent surges of sugar which reach the blood from eating and drinking throughout the day and between meals. For instance, five sugared cups of tea a day if taken for fifty years will have stimulated the pancreas 91,000 times. The pancreas, as a result, eventually becomes exhausted and ceases to produce sufficient insulin to convert into a digestible form, all the sugar ingested as this continues to be absorbed into the blood from the stomach and intestine. The unconverted (and therefore unusable) sugar is eventually excreted in the urine but not before it has caused damage which eventually leads to serious forms of ill-health such as increased liability to infection, gangrene and blindness. Yet this type of diabetes can be readily controlled by a timely reduction in the amounts of sugar consumed, particularly when accompanied by a simultaneous increase in the proportion of high-fibre food. This effectively reduces the need for rapid insulin production, because dietary fibre slows absorption from the intestines.

Atherosclerosis: This disease comes on gradually and insidiously, as excess fat in the form of cholesterol-plaques begins to be deposited along the arteries, particularly where there is a bend. Progressively the artery closes, restricting the blood flow and the blood pressure increases to keep up an adequate supply. The usually smooth glistening lining of the vessels becomes uneven and roughened; the vessel walls lose their usual elasticity and become hard and brittle. Eventually the damaged, brittle vessel-wall will crack with escape of blood into the surrounding tissues.

A Stroke When a blood vessel ruptures in the brain, which happens frequently in persons with raised blood pressure, they suffer what is called a stroke, and the patient becomes paralysed as a result of the greatly increased pressure by the escaped blood on the highly specialised nervous tissues, the compressed portion of the brain no longer being able to execute its function. The gravity of the condition will depend principally on the actual site of the leak, the size of the haemorrhage and amount of brain tissue that has been invaded and damaged by the escaped blood. A stroke can also be caused by a blood clot (called brain infarct) frequently in conjunction with a detached fragment of cholesterol floating in it. Together they lodge in and block a narrowed blood vessel in the brain. In obese people, owing to the increased stickiness of the blood-clotting cells (platelets) this is an all too frequent complication. When it happens the section of the brain, deprived by the clot of the oxygen-carrying blood supply, perishes because it cannot survive and function without oxygen and in time scar tissue will form.

Heart Disease The main cause of heart disease, which annually claims over 200,000 lives in the UK, many of them only in their early forties, is to be found in the previously described silting-up and eventual blockage of blood vessels. With this disease it is the coronary arteries (that carry oxygen to the heart) which are affected. The body's fantastic ability to adapt and protect itself enables tiny new blood vessels to grow around the obstruction in the artery and keep a limited blood flow going. Without adequate oxygen the heart-beat becomes erratic and the heart will eventually stop beating altogether. Such heart "arrest" (coronary thrombosis) occurs predominantly in over-nourished people who, despite not being engaged in strenuous physical exercise or vigorous sporting activities, continue to include the usual generous amounts of fat and sugar in their daily food and thus eat meals which should be reserved solely for dedicated athletes in full hard training.

Since the only function of fats and sugar in the body, as already mentioned, is that of providing fuel for muscular activity, in the absence of such physical exertion it is inevitable that the surplus energy will not only tend to clog-up the arteries but, when stored as fat, will also contribute to a corresponding gain in weight.

The vicious circle is that being too heavy discourages one from taking vigorous exercise, and physical inactivity further encourages the deposition of fat and yet a further increase in weight.

Cancer Basically, the destructive process within us that we call cancer can originate in the body only because of the remarkable ability of living tissue to compensate for abuse, injury or damage, by initiating an acceleration of cellular activity thereby forming new tissues with which to repair the damage. Normally, this is a highly orderly and strict time-limited process.

However, when the factors causing the abuse, injury or damage, such as dietary excesses, addiction to cigarettes or over-consumption of alcohol are repetitive, that is when they continue to operate regularly, day after day and year after year, then the body's attempts at repair will eventually become disorderly and will escalate into unrestrained cellular activity finally ending in uncontrolled growth: cancer.

Further Reading

Diet and Nutrition

The Low Fat Way to Health and Longer Life *by Lester Morrison*

Vitamin E for Ailing and Healthy Hearts *by Wilfred Shute*

Pure, White and Deadly *by G. Yudkin*

Natural Health, Sugar and the Criminal Mind *by J.I. Rodale*

Supernutrition by Richard Passwater

The Saccharine Disease *by Thomas Cleave*

Cooking for your Life *by Marlene Pentecost*

The Pritkin Program for Diet and Exercise *by Nathan Pritkin*

Ecology of Food and Nutrition *by Michele Brenner*

A Macrobiotic Approach to Cancer *by Sean McLean*

Human Nutrition and Dietetics *by Sir Stanley Davidson*

Don't Forget Fibre in Your Diet *by Dennis Burkitt*

Calories and Nutrition *by Arnold Bender*

The Complete Scarsdale Medical Diet *by Herman Tarnover*

The Health Revolution *by Ross Hone*

Food is Your Best Medicine *by H.G. Bieler*

The F-Plan Diet *by Audrey Eyton*

Exercise

Aeorobics *by Kenneth Cooper*

Total Fitness in 30 Minutes a Week *by L. Morhouse*

The Physiological Effect of Exercise Programs on Adults
by Thomas Cureton

Prevention of Ischaemic Heart Disease *by Wilhelm Raab*
Antibodies and Immunity *by G.J. Nossal*
You Can Fight for Your Life *by Ray Roseman*
Getting Well Again *by Stephanie Simonton*
Man the Unknown *by Alexis Carrel*
Health and Light *by John Ott*

Bloodstream

Blood the Paramount Humour *by Earle Hackett*
Blood, Micro-Rheology Viscosity Factors in Blood Flow
by Leopold Dintenfas
Rheology of Blood in Diagnostic and Preventive Medicine
by Leopold Dintenfas

Cancer Prevention

Medical Radiation Biology *by E. Ellinger*
Cancer — A Disease of Civilisation *by Vilhjamur Stephansson*
Cancer — The Facts *by Sir Ronald Bodley Scott*
Physiology of Cancer *by Albert Tannenbaum*
A Time to Heal *by Joseph Issels*
A Cancer Therapy — The Result of 50 Cases *by Max Gerson*
Has Dr. Max Gerson A True Cancer Cure *by J. Shaught*
Cancer and Cure — A Doctor's Study *by Eva Hill*
Preventing Cancer *by Elizabeth Whelan*
How to Avoid Cancer *by Jan de Winter*
The Causes of Cancer *by Richard Doll*

Epidemiology

Health Conditions and Disease Incidence among the Eskimos
of Labrador *by Samuel Hutton*
Health Secrets of Hunza *by Renee Taylor*
Hunza Land *by Allen E. Bank*
Primitive Life Keeps Tribesmen's Hearts Strong *by P.F. Sinnoth*

Emotional Stress

Rodale's System for Mental Power and Natural Health
by J.I. Rodale
Stress Without Distress *by Hans Selye*
Faith Healing *by Louie Rose*
Mind and Body *by Stephen Black*
The Healing Factor *by Irwin Stone*

Preventive Medicine

The Wheel of Health *by G.T. Wrench*
Lifestyles, Major Risk Factors, Proof and Public Policy
by Jeremiah Stamler
Anatomy of Illness *by Norman Cousins*
Type "A" Behaviour and Your Heart *by Meyer Friedman*
Confessions of a Medical Heretic *by Robert S. Mendelsohn*
The Body is the Hero *by Ronald Glaser*
Youth in Old Age *by Alexander Leaf*
Its Your Body — A Woman's Guide to Gynaecology
by Niels Laverson
Live Longer Now *by Nathan Pritkin*

INDEX